Khaled Sultan

Key Findings in Veterinary Parasitology I. Veterinary Helminthology

Khaled Sultan

Key Findings in Veterinary Parasitology I. Veterinary Helminthology

Platyhelminthes I. Digenetic Trematoda & Cestoda

LAP LAMBERT Academic Publishing

Imprint

Any brand names and product names mentioned in this book are subject to trademark, brand or patent protection and are trademarks or registered trademarks of their respective holders. The use of brand names, product names, common names, trade names, product descriptions etc. even without a particular marking in this work is in no way to be construed to mean that such names may be regarded as unrestricted in respect of trademark and brand protection legislation and could thus be used by anyone.

Cover image: www.ingimage.com

Publisher:
LAP LAMBERT Academic Publishing
is a trademark of
International Book Market Service Ltd., member of OmniScriptum Publishing Group
17 Meldrum Street, Beau Bassin 71504, Mauritius

ISBN: 978-3-659-54992-2

Copyright © Khaled Sultan
Copyright © 2014 International Book Market Service Ltd., member of OmniScriptum Publishing Group

Key Findings in Veterinary Parasitology

I. Veterinary Helminthology

Platyhelminthes

I. Digenetic Trematoda & Cestoda

By

Khaled Sultan

Lecturer in Parasitology,
Faculty of Veterinary Medicine,
Kafrelsheikh University,
33516 Kafr El-Sheik, Egypt

About the Author

Khaled Sultan received his Ph.D. in Parasitology from Kafrelsheikh University in 2012. The author did research for his doctoral degree at Yamguchi University (Laboratory of Veterinary Parasitology) in Japan. He is currently a lecturer in Parasitology at Kafrelsheikh University. The author has published actively his works in international scientific journals. The main focus of his study is the exploration and the identification of parasites in ruminants and wild animals, using both morphological and molecular approaches.

About this book

This book is a handbook for students that offers concise information on digenetic trematodes and cestodes that infect domestic and wild animals. It is useful particularly for undergraduates in the fields who have taken or are currently taking Parasitology or Zoology course, and for the general audience who have interests in Parasitology. It is not intended to be a comprehensive textbook in the field of Parasitology. It is hoped that this text will be helpful to understand the outline of the parasites and their diseases.

ACKNOWLEDGEMENTS

Praise to God (ALLAH) the merciful, for His blessing and His grace. Words cannot express my true feelings and my thanks for all the friends who helped me through this work, for their valuable support, interest and suggestions for improvements. Also, for her valuable help in English language edition of this book; I would like to thank Dr. Agatha Bardoel, a science writer at Natioanl Laboratory, Tennessee, USA.

I am grateful to my dear Professor. Hiroshi Sato, Yamaguchi University, Japan for the scientific revision of this work.

This work is dedicated to my parents, to my wife and to my lovely daughters.

K. Sultan

CONTENTS

	Page
INTRODUCTION	4
Platyhelminthes	7
Class TREMATODA	7
Class CESTODA	32
REFERENCES	57

INTRODUCTION:

Veterinary Parasitology is the study of parasites that invade animals, and focuses largely on the relationship between parasites and their larger, animal hosts. Parasites in domestic animals (livestock and pet animals) as well as in wildlife animals are considered here.

A "parasite" is defined as a pathogen, a "eukaryotic organism", that simultaneously derives sustenance from and injures its host. These small organisms both gain benefits and cause harm to the larger organisms (i.e. the host) that they invade.

The biological relationships among living organisms may be classified concisely as follows:

1. Symbiosis (Mutualism): This refers to two unlike organisms living together, to afford such advantages as protection to one and nutrient supply to the other, or two organisms of neutral relationships with neither benefit or harm to each other.

2. Commensalism: This refers to a symbiotic relationship between two organisms living together in neutrality, i.e., with one way benefit such as protection or nutrient supply.

3- Parasitism: A non-mutual, symbiotic relationship in which one organism (the parasite), lives at the expense of the other (the host). The parasite depends on the host for its survival and gains benefits that may cause harm to the host.

Parasites may be classified into multiple categories, depending on many factors. Here we restrict our discussion of these organisms to:

I. Their habitat or mode of development:

1. Endoparasites: a parasite living inside the body of a host, such as Fasciola spp.

2. Ectoparasite: a parasite living on the outside of a host body, such as lice.

II. Their life cycle:

1. Obligate parasites: To complete their development and to propagate, these require a host at almost all stages of their life cycle. An example is liver and blood flukes.

2. Facultative parasites: These may exist freely in a living state or they may become parasitic under certain circumstances. Freeliving protozoans such as *Naegleria fowleri* and *Acanthamoeba* spp can also cause miningoencephalitis in human beings.

3. Accidental or Incidental parasites: These establish and continue their life cycle in a host in which they are not ordinarily found. Sheep bot larvae, "*Oestrus ovis*", are an example found in humans.

4. Permanent parasites: These remain on or in the body of the host for its entire life cycle. Sucking lice are an example.

5. Temporary parasites: These live on the host for a short period of their life cycle, such as fleas.

We turn now to the "host". The host may be conveniently classified according to its role in the life cycle of the parasite:

1. Definitive or final host: These are hosts in which the sexual maturity and reproduction of the parasite takes place e.g. Ruminants for *Fasciola* parasite; dogs for *Echinococcus granulosus*.

2. Intermediate host: These are hosts in which the asexual phase of the parasite life cycle occurs and the larval stage develops, e.g. in the case of *Fasciola* as parasite and the *Lymnea* snail as intermediate host is a good example.

3. Paratenic host: These are hosts in which the parasite does not develop to its later stages. However, the parasite remains alive and it is able to infect another susceptible host. Rodents for *Toxocara cati* (a species of nematodes).

4. Reservoir hosts: These allow a parasite's life cycle to continue and to become a source of infection. Protozoan parasites *Leishmania* spp. infecting human beings takes dogs as a reservoir host.

5. Vectors: These are responsible for transmitting a parasite from one host to another, such as mosquitoes that transmit malaria pathogen *Plasmodium* spp. to humans.

Vectors may be subclassified into:

a. Biologic vectors that transmit a parasite and within which the parasite can change in shape or number during its development, such as *Plasmodium* spp. in mosquitoes
b. Mechanical vectors that transport a parasite without changing it, as a flagellated protozoan "*Trypanosoma evnasi*" can be transported by the *Tabanus* fly .

6. Carrier hosts: A type of host that harbors a parasite without any signs and symptoms, for example, a bull for a flagellated protozoan *Tritrichominas foetus*.

We define a few terms of importance in this book:
Exposure: This refers to the opportunity of an infective agent "the infective stage of parasites" is inoculated orally or entering a host by another ways.

Infection: This refers to the establishment of the infective agent (the parasite) in the host.

It should be noted that "infect' and 'infection' are used to describe the invasion of a host by a parasite. These terms are now applicable not only to virus, bacteria and protozoa, but also to helminths. The terms "infest" and "infestation" however may not be applied to an invasion by helminths, but used frequently for the infection process of ectoparasies.

Incubation period: This refers to the period of time that elapses between the occurrence of an infection and the manifestation of symptoms or of clinical signs.

Autoinfection: In a broad sense, this occurs when an infected individual is itself the source of the infection with which it is afflicted. Exactly or strictly saying, some kinds of parasites produce their descendents in the same individual without development outside the body; e.g. *Strongyloides stercoralis, Cryptosporidium* spp., etc.

Super-infection or Hyper-infection: This refers to the recurrence of infection by the same species in a host that is already infected or has been previously infected. This may result in a further, massive infection.

Sources of infection may be:

1. Contaminated soil and water; e.g. *Ancylostoma* and *Schistosoma*.

2. Contaminated food; e.g. *Fasciola, Taenia solium*.

3. Arthropods; e.g. *Dipylidium caninum*.

4. Animals may be a direct source of infection; e.g. *Tritrichomonas foetus*.

General modes of transmission may be:

1. Mouth (per os, ingestion); e.g. *Fasciola, Taenia solium*.

2. Skin penetration (per cutaneous); e.g. *Schistosoma, Ancylostoma*.

3. Arthropods; e.g. *Plasmodium*.

4. Congenital transmission (vertical); e.g. *Toxoplasma gondii*.

5. Transplacental; e.g. *Toxocara canis*.

5. Transmammmary; e.g. *Toxocara cati*.

6. Inhalation; e.g. *Giardia deuodenalis*.

7. Sexual intercourse (Venereal); e.g. *Tritrichomonas foetus*

We may divide **Parasitology** into three main branches, according to the type of parasites with which we are dealing: "**Helminthology**" (that field deals with metazoan endoparasites such as flukes, tapeworms, nematodes and acanthocephalans), "**Entomology**" (that field deals with arthropods), and "**Protozoology**" (that field deals with protozoa, unicellular enkaryotes).

Note that the words "**Helminthology** is the study of endoparasitic worms. Knowledge of parasitic worms is very ancient. The name is derived from the Greek word "HELMINTHO", which refers to worms, and "LOGOS" which means "word". Helminths "worms, Vermes" are multicellular invertebrate animals. Helminths include Nematoda (roundworms), Nematomorpha (hairworms), Platyhelminthes (flatworms), Acanthocephala (thorny-headed worms), and Annelida (earthworms and leeches).

Platyhelminthes "Flatworm"

The Greek name Platyhelminthes is composed of two words, "platy" which means flat, and "helminthes" which means worms.

This phylum contains members of the bilaterally symmetrical "their sides a mirror image of each other", of the acoelomates (having no body cavity), and of the compressed dorsoventral worms. They have simple digestive system (trematodes) or none (cestodes), and no specific circulatory or respiratory systems. Nutrition absorption occurs mainly through diffusion.

Platyhelminthes comprise four classes:

1) **Turbellaria**. These are mainly free living non parasites.

2) **Monogena**: These are mainly occurring in fishes and cold blooded animals.

3) **Digenea "Trematoda" "Flukes"**.

Members of the class Trematoda are unsegmented flatworms.

The class Trematoda may be classified into three main subclasses, according to the nature and number of hosts required to complete the life cycle:

The subclass "Aspidogastrea", of which most species of this subclass require one host to complete the life cycle. These are parasites that may be found in turtles and fishes.

The "Digenea", which require at least two hosts to complete the life cycle. The intermediate host is usually a mollusk (a snail).

These digenetic trematodes are parasites that occur in nearly all vertebrates, including domestic animals, wild animals, fish, and humans.

The third subclass into which the class Trematoda may be classified is the subclass "Didymozoidea." These are parasites found in fish, and we currently have little data on their life cycle.

They exhibit great variation in shape and size. With the exception of *Schistosoma* spp. (blood flukes), most flukes are flattened dorsoventrally, have a blind alimentary tract (ceca), and usually two suckers for attachment, they are hermaphrodites.

During the life cycle, adult flukes produce eggs that pass out from the final host with its excreta. The larval stage develops in the intermediate host, usually a snail, developing from miracidium to sporocysts, redia and finally cercariae. In a few species, e.g. *Heterophyes* and *Dicrocoelium*, a second intermediate host is required. With the exception of *Shcistosoma* spp., the infection of the final host occurs by ingestion of the infective encysted metacercaria, where the metacercaria develops to the adult stage in the specific organ.

In these worms, the adult flukes possess two suckers (oral and ventral) for attachment. The oral sucker at the anterior end surrounds the mouth (oral opening) and the ventral sucker presents on the ventral side. In some species, another sucker may be present, surrounding the common genital pore, called the "genital sucker" e.g. *Heterophyes* spp. In some species, e.g. *Echinostoma*, an additional specialized spiny structure "head collar", is present and surrounds the oral opening.

The body surface "tegument" is protective and absorptive, and is often covered with minute spines. The muscles lie immediately below the tegument. There is no body cavity "i.e. acolemate" and the organs are packed in a parenchyma.

The digestive system is simple; the oral opening leads into a pharynx (which may surround the esophagus completely, partially, or be absent), then into an esophagus and then into a pair of branched intestinal ceca that end blindly (i.e. there is no anal opening). The branching of the intestinal ceca facilitates the diffusion of nutrients to the body of the fluke. The digestion process is usually extracellular.

The excretory system features a large number of highly specialized units called flame cells (flame bulbs; protonephiridium), that impel waste metabolic products along a system of tubules that then join and open to the exterior.

The nervous system of adult flukes is simple, and consists of a pair of longitudinal nerve cords that connect transversely with ring commissures (ganglia). There are three main longitudinal nerve trunks (dorsal, lateral, and ventral) and these arise from the anterior part (cephalic ganglia) and continue to emanate to the rest of the body posteriorly. To complete the life cycle, the larval stages (e.g. miracidia and cercariae) of the flukes also have specialized sensory organs (e.g. eyespots) to respond to certain stimuli. Most flukes are hermaphrodite with the exception of *Schistosoma* spp. and both cross- and self-fertilization may occur.

The male reproductive system in most flukes consists firstly of a pair of testes. There may be as many as 6 to 9 testes in some species, such as the schistosomes. Each testes leads into a vas deferens; these join to enter the cirrus sac, which contains a seminal vesicle (for sperm storage). The cirrus sac contains the cirrus, a primitive retractile penis that terminates at the genital opening, a shallow genital atrium. The genital atrium in most flukes is typically present in the midventral surface, anterior to the ventral sucker. The male ejaculatory duct is surrounded by the prostate gland cells, which may form the pars prositatica.

How the two testes are positioned relative to each other varies by species. When the two testes are arranged parallel to the vertical axis (i.e. one above the other), this is called "tandem". The arrangement may also be "oblique" or "horizontal". The shape of the testes varies according to the species; they may be branched, lobed or smooth. The female system in most flukes consists of a single ovary leading into an oviduct, which is expanded to form the seminal receptacle; a vestigial vagina (Luarer's canal) may be present.

The ovum (egg) requires a yolk from the secretion of the vitelline gland. The vitelline glands (= vitelleria) typically present in two groups laterally and there are networks of ducts that connect these glands to a common vitelline duct which joins the oviduct. An ootype is formed as a result of the expansion of the oviduct. Another type of specialized gland called "Mehils' glands" is present and surrounds the ootype. Beyond the ootype, the uterus is formed. As the egg passes along the uterus, the shell becomes hardened and toughened and is finally extruded through the genital opening adjacent to the ventral sucker. The mature egg is usually yellow because of the tanned protein shell. Most fluke species eggs have an operculum.

Digenea life cycle:

It is remarkable that by means of asexual development within the intermediate snail host, one trematode egg may develop into hundreds that successfully achieve the subsequent developmental stages. The adult flukes are always oviparous (egg-laying). Most of fluke eggs have an operculum (a structure at one pole of the egg) that resembles the air sac in the eggs in hens. Within the egg, the embryo develops into a pyriform, ciliated organism, called a miracidium. Under stimulus (such as chemical or phototropic stimuli), the miracidium releases an enzyme that then attacks the cement material that holds the operculum in place. The operculum then can open and the miracidium can be released. The miracidium, typically swims in the water by its cilia (except those of Dicrocoliedae). It does not feed and for its further development it must find a suitable snail host, within a few hours. Miracidia penetrate the soft tissues of the snail, aided by a cytolytic enzyme.

If the miracidium fails to find a host, they die. Subsequently the cilia are lost and the miracidium develops into an elongated sac-like structure called "the sporocyst", and this contains a number of germinal cells. These cells develop into the "redia", the next developmental stage. The redia is more highly developed, have a muscular pharynx and a simple gut.

From the germinal cells of the rediae, the final stages arise. The cercaria, is a simple structure with a body part and tail. The body part bears suckers that resemble that of the adult, a simple digestive tract, and specialized glands "penetration glands" that aid in the penetration of the host tissue.

Cercariae emerge actively from the snails. Typically the cercariae swim for some time, utilizing a film of water, and within an hour they may attach themselves to a hard object, such as stones or vegetation, or penetrate fish or other amphibian tissues as in case of *Heterophyes heterophyes*, shed their tails and become encysted. This stage is called encysted metacercaria. It is the common infective stage of flukes. Encysted metacercariae have great potential for survival and can live for months. Once they are ingested by a susceptible final host, the outer cyst wall is removed mechanically; intestinal secretions remove the inner cyst wall. The emergent juvenile fluke then penetrates the intestine and migrates to its habitat, where after weeks it becomes an adult.

Digenea classification:

There are thousands of digenetic trematodes of veterinary and medical importance. Here are the most important.

Family FASCIOLIDAE

These are large leaf-shaped flukes, featuring an anterior end that is typically lengthened into a cone. An anterior sucker is located at the tip of the cone, and a ventral sucker is positioned at the shoulder level. The tegument is spiny.

Within this family, there are three important genera, ***Fasciola***, ***Fascioloides*** and ***Fasciolopsis***.

Genus *Fasciola*

The members of genus *Fasciola* are commonly known as **liver flukes**, named after the organ in the host where they are found. Liver flukes cause a disease condition called **fascioliasis, distomatosis, liver rot**. These flukes cause considerable morbidity and mortality in ruminants all over the world, and can infect humans as final host "i.e. zoonotic helminths".

Fascioliasis is a disease that is prevalent worldwide; the two most important species responsible for the disease are *F. hepatica*, found in Europe and in other temperate-subtropical areas and at cooler, high altitudes in the tropics and subtropics; and *F. gigantica*, which predominates in Africa and in tropical Asia, Southeast Asia, the Pacific regions, and some parts of North America. Another form called "**the hybrid form, aspermic *Fasciola* sp.**" has now been scientifically documented, it is present mainly in East Asia including Japan, Korea and China, South East Asia and Egypt, and is thought to be the result of hyberdization between the two earlier *Fasciola* species. This hybrid form possesses the morphological appearance of *F. hepatica* and shares the genetic makeup of *F. gigantica*.

Hosts: Most mammals may be final host; particularly domestic and wild ruminants including sheep, goats, cattle, buffaloes, camels, and deer. Sheep and cattle are the most ubiquitous host. Other vulnerable animal species include equines, rabbits, pigs and monkeys.
Intermediate hosts: The most common intermediate hosts are snails of the genus *Lymnaea* e.g. *L. truncatula*, an amphibious snail with a wide distribution throughout the world. Other snails may act as intermediate hosts, e.g. *Fossoria*, and the snail species may vary with geographical differences.

Habitat: Adult *Fasciola* spp. are found in the bile ducts and the immature flukes in the liver parenchyma of their definitive hosts.

Distribution: Worldwide.

Identification: Fully mature *Fasciola* in the bile ducts are typically leaf-shaped and grey-brown in color. The mature liver flukes are large flukes, and the size varies. *F. hepatica* is typically about 2- 5 cm long by 0.6-1.3 cm wide. *F. gigantica* is larger and may grow to 7.6 cm in length. The anterior end of *F. hepatica* is conical and is marked by shoulders that are distinct from the body.

In *F. gigantica* the two sides of the body are generally parallel and the shoulders are less distinct. In the anterior part of the fluke, oral and ventral suckers are closely adjacent and are visible to the naked eye as small orifices. The ventral sucker is positioned at shoulder level. The tegument is spiny. The digestive system features a well developed pharynx and the branched intestinal ceca are long. There are two testes, tandem in position and branched. The ovary is also branched and anterior to the testes. The vitelline glands are well developed and are presented in two groups, almost filling the lateral sides. The uterus is relatively short.

The egg is oval, operculated, unembryonared, golden-yellow in color, and large (about 130-190 μm long by 70-100 μm wide), containing an ovum and vitelline cells.

Fasciola life cycle

Eggs passed in the feces of the final host (e.g. ruminants), enter the fresh water canals, develop, and hatch, releasing the motile ciliated stage "miracidium" in about 9 days. Miracidium survival is dependent on environmental temperature; the optimum temperature for its survival is about 22°C (15-25 °C).

Miracidia have a short life span. Within a few hours, they must enter the intermediate snail host, in which their development proceeds by asexual multiplication through sporocyst, and redia, and finally cercariae.

The cercaria leaves the snail host and moves through water by the aid of a tail, attaching itself finally to a firm surface (e.g. nearby stones, and plants including watercress and other vegetables). There it encysts and forms the infective metacercariae.

The life cycle of *Fasciola* from the miracidium to encysted metacercaria is about 6-7 weeks in length in favorable conditions (with a temperature of about 20-25 °C), but it may extend to several months in adverse environmental conditions such as low temperature (below 12°C).

The infection of a snail with one miracidium can produce more than 600 metacercariae. Encysted metacercariae ingested by the final host excyst in the small intestine, penetrate the gut wall, migrate cross the peritoneum, and again penetrate the liver capsule. The young flukes migrate through the liver parenchyma for some 5-6 weeks and then enter the small bile ducts, where they further move to the larger ducts and there mature. The prepatent period is about 2 months. The whole life cycle of *Fasciola* spp. is about 14-23 weeks.

There are three main factors influencing the epidemiology of *Fasciola*.

1. Availability of the intermediate snail host.

2. Temperature.

3. Moisture.

These three factors are essential to ensure the life cycle and to produce an outbreak of fascioliasis.

Pathogenesis and clinical signs

These vary according to the phase of development in the liver and the species of the host. Fasciolosis may be acute, sub-acute, or chronic.

1. The acute form of fascioliasis:

This occurs 2-6 weeks after the ingestion of large numbers of encysted metacercariae, typically more 2000. The acute stage of the disease is characterized by the severe hemorrhage that results when the young flukes migrating in the liver parenchyma rupture the blood vessels of that organ, causing severe injury. The main clinical picture for acute fascioliasis is sudden death, which usually occurs in sheep flocks during autumn and early winter. Some sheep within the affected flock may show weakness, with pale mucus membranes and palpable enlarged livers, accompanied by abdominal pain and ascitis. Note that the acute phase may be prolonged and may turn into a subacute or even a chronic form. The main gross findings at necropsy are in the liver; typically this is enlarged and hemorrhagic with the tracts of migrating immature flukes. The surface, particularly over the ventral lobe, is frequently covered with fibrinous exudate. Subcapsular hemorrhage is also common and a quantity of blood-stained fluid may be present in the abdominal cavity. Taking a slice of the affected liver and the immersion of these parts in warm water will reveal the presence of the juvenile flukes.

Black disease is a syndrome that occasionally occurs with acute fasciolisais outbreaks, as a result of the complicated infections with anaerobic bacterium *Clostridium novyi*. Black disease is usually fatal due to the toxins that this type of bacteria releases.

2. The sub-acute form of fascioliasis:

This form of the disease results from the ingestion of a lesser number of the encysted metacercariae (approximately 500-1500) and its effects occur over a longer period (typically 6-10 weeks after ingestion). It also manifests in the host animal in the late autumn and winter.

During this period, some migrated flukes reach the bile ducts and mature into adults, while other, younger flukes are still in the migratory phase, causing hepatic lesions similar to those of the acute form.

At necropsy, the liver is found to be enlarged with numerous necrotic or hemorrhagic tunnels. Subcapsular hepatic hemorrhages are typically present. The clinical picture of the sub-acute form presents as a rapid loss of body condition, marked pale mucous membranes, and an enlarged and palpable liver. The characteristic sub-mandibular "bottle-jaw" or facial edema and ascites may be present. These signs are a result of hepatic lesions which subsequently lead to severe hemorrhagic anemia, with severe hypoalbuminanemia (a notable decrease of albumin in the blood) and esinophilia. If not treated, the animal loses its productivity and a high mortality rate may occur in affected herds. Clinical signs appear 1-2 weeks prior to death.

3. The chronic form of fascioliasis:

This form of the disease is usually seen in late winter and early spring. It is the most common form of fascioliasis and particularly in large ruminants. It occurs over a period of 4-5 months after the ingestion of some 200-500 encysted metacercariae. Clinically, it presents mainly as a progressive loss of fitness, a loss of productivity, emaciation, pale mucous membranes, submandibular edema (**bottle-jaw**), and ascites.

A moderate to severe loss of animal productivity occurs. These signs occur as a result of anemia and hypoalbuminanemia, due to liver lesions and feeding flukes. When the blood is examined, the anaemia is found to be hypochromic and macrocytic, with marked esinophilia. In necropsy, the liver is found to have a pale color and a firm consistency. Microscopically, the affected liver shows hepatic fibrosis; hyperplastic cholangitis and egg's granuloma may be evident. Calcification of the bile ducts and enlargement of the gallbladder may be noticed.

A disease called "**Halzon or pharyngeal fascioliasis**" in humans was initially reported as a result of eating uncooked raw animal liver that had been infected with *Fasciola*.

However subsequent work now attributes the incident to the ingestion of a nymphal stage of another arthropod parasite, *Lingatula serrata*.

Diagnosis of fascioliasis

To successfully diagnose fascioliasis, a step by step examination is done through:

1. Case history (season, grazing history, snail population within the locality, etc.)

2. Clinical signs.

3. Fecal examination (to detect characteristic *Fasciola* eggs by the sedimentation method).

4. Hematological test (to demonstrate anemia, hypoproteinemia, esinophillia, liver enzymes titer).

5. Serological tests (e.g. Enzyme Linked Immunosorbent Assay "ELISA" to detect specific antibodies to *Fasciola*).

6. Necropsy procedures, if available. Usually this step follows a diagnosis of acute fascioliasis in sheep.

Treatment of fasciolisais

Several drugs are now available for treatment of the *Fasciola* infection, including triclabendazole, rafoxanide, closantel and nitroxynil. Praziquantel is not fully effective against *Fasciola*.

Triclabendazole is the drug of choice for both treatment and control of fascioliasis, given in a single dose of 10 mg/kg body weight.

It is well-known that triclabendazole is effective against mature and immature flukes, while the other drugs are effective only in adult animals. A single dose of triclabendazole, accompanied by a good management, should be a sufficient treatment. This may be followed by a second dose (and even a third dose) at a 2-3 weeks interval, to achieve the total removal of a fluke burden from the affected flock.

Control of fascioliasis

Control of this parasite may be approached in two ways:

A. Control of the intermediate snail population, through strategies such as biological control (e.g. rearing snail-predator fish in water channels), chemicals (e.g. copper sulphate or any other molluscicides), and mechanical (e.g. proper drainage and improving the capacity of water channels).

B. Prophylactic anthelmintics treatment. The same group of anthelmintics used for treatment can be used to reduce egg output and as a prophylactic for susceptible herds in areas where the parasite is endemic.

Genus *Fascioloides*

Fascioloides magna

This is the **deer liver fluke, [or] large American liver fluke**.

This parasite is found mainly in ruminants and particularly in wild deer but it can significantly affect other animals, such as pigs, horses, and rodents. It is found in North and Central America, expanding its distribution recently in several European countries. Morphologically, *Fascioloides magna* is a very large fluke measuring up to 7 cm (usually 3.5-5 cm long by 1.7- 3.2 cm wide). It has no anterior cone. The life cycle resembles that of *Fasciola* species, and several lymnaeid snails appear to be the intermediate host. In deer and cattle, the parasite, on reaching the liver, may cause hepatic damage, but it rapidly becomes encapsulated. In sheep, encapsulation of the parasite does not occur, and as a result, damage to the liver can be severe, even fatal.

Genus *Fasciolopsis*

Fasciolopsis buski

This is a neglected parasite found in humans, but it can also infect a range of animals, including swines, equines, bovines and ovines. It is prevalent in South East Asia. It is commonly called the "giant intestinal fluke", because it is an exceptionally large parasitic fluke. Its length is variable from 2 to 7.5 cm and it can have a width of 2.5 cm. It can be distinguished from other members of family Fasciolidae by a lack of cephalic cone or "shoulders" and by its unbranched ceca. The life cycle is much similar to other members of the family.

Family DICROCOELIDAE

Genus: *Dicrocoelium*

This parasite is typically described as "**lancet-like flukes, lanceolate-liver flukes, small liver flukes**" due to its small size and its characteristic body shape which resembles a lancet or a blade.

Hosts: It has a wide range of hosts but it mainly infects domestic and wild ruminants, including sheep, cattle and deer. It can also infect humans. Intermediate hosts: Two are required to complete the life cycle. The first are land snails of many genera (e.g. ***Zebrina*** spp., ***Hellicela*** spp.); the second, ants of the genus *Formica*.

Habitat: Adults inhabit the bile ducts and the gall bladder.

Distribution: Worldwide.

Species: *Dicrocoelium dendriticum* is the most common species worldwide; other species such as *D. chinenses* and *D. hospes* are also endemic in Asia and Africa, respectively.

Dicrocoelium dendriticum **identification**: This fluke are about 1 cm long by 0.25 cm wide, with a body that has pointed ends and is semitransparent. Adults have an oral and ventral sucker, the latter being larger, and a digestive system with two long intestinal ceca. The testes are lobated, lie in tandem position and a single ovary is located posterior to these. The long uterus is complexly folded, is filled with brown eggs, and it occupies a posterior half of the body behind the ovary. Vitelleria present in the lateral sides and are extracecal in the middle part. The cuticle is smooth. The egg is small, approximately 45 by 30 µm, is dark brown in color and is operculated, usually with a flattened side. The egg contains a miracidium when passed in the feces.

Dicrocoelium dendriticum life cycle

The egg hatches after it is ingested by a first intermediate host, in which two generations of sporocysts develop without redia formation, which then produce cercariae. The cercariae are expelled from the snail host in cercariae masses (which contain about 5000 cercariae), cemented together by slime. These masses are called "**slime-balls**". The development within the snail host takes from 3-4 months. The slime balls of cercariae are ingested by the second intermediate host, in which they develop to metacercariac, mainly in the body cavity and occasionally in the brain.

The development in the second intermediate host takes from 1-2 months. The infected ants that contain metacercaria are then ingested by a final host.

In the final host, the metacercariae hatch in the small intestine and the young flukes migrate up the main bile duct and then the smaller ducts in the liver; there is no hepatic migration, such as occurs in *Fasciola*. In the final host, the prepatent period is 2 months. The flukes are long-lived and can survive in the final host for several years.

Dicrocoelium dendriticum pathogenesis and clinical signs

Dicrocoelium dendriticum infection is largely without clinical signs, due to the fact that the liver is not as severely affected as it is in *Fasciola*. However, when the infection is severe and thousands of the lancet liver flukes are present, cirrhosis of the liver and bile ducts may occur, resulting in anemia, edema, emaciation, and loss of production.

Dicrocoelium dendriticum epidemiology

Three factors control the epidemiology of *Dicrocoleium*;

1. The intermediate hosts are land snails and ants.

2. The eggs are persistent for long periods.

3. Some environmental and ecological factors exist, such as alkalinity of the soil.

These factors play the key role in *D. dentriticum* infection and epidemiology and create the difficulties in attempting to control the infection.

Dicrocoelium dendriticum diagnosis, treatment and control

A diagnosis is based mainly on fecal examination to identify the eggs and on the necropsy findings. Other serological techniques may be applied to detect anti-*Dicrocoelium* antibodies. Drugs such as netobimin, albendazole, thiabendazole, and tricalbendazole are also effective, but at a higher dosage than is recommended to treat other helminth infection. The successful control of this parasite depends mainly on the regular anthelmintics treatment of infected and susceptible animals.

Genus: *Eurytrema*

The most common species is *Eurytrema pancreaticum*, which inhabits the pancreatic ducts of ruminants especially in South-East Asia.

Morphologically, adult flukes are small, 8-16 mm long and 5-8 mm wide. They are thick, with a spiny tegument, and have two suckers, of which the oral sucker is larger than the ventral one. The digestive system, intestinal ceca, is simple. The testes are lobed, just behind the ventral sucker. The ovary is small, lobed, and posterior to the testes. The vitelline gland locates laterally at the mid-body. The uterus is long and coiled, occupying the posterior half of the body. The eggs are similar to those of *D. dendriticum*.

Similarly to *D. dendriticum*, *Eurytrema pancreaticum* has two intermediate hosts, a terrestrial (land) snail, followed by grasshoppers. Infection of the final host is by ingestion of the grasshopper and the fluke migrates from the small intestine to the pancreatic ducts, the final site in the pancreas.

If the infection is light it can be without symptoms. In cases of heavy infection, fibrosis and atrophy of the pancreas may occur.

Family OPISTHORCHIDAE

Genus *Opisthorchis*
These are human liver flukes that infect millions of people, mainly in Southeast Asia and Europe.

Species: *Opisthorchis viverrini* (**Southeast Asian liver fluke**) and *O. felineus* (**cat liver fluke**).

Hosts: Mainly human but can infect cats.
Intermediate hosts: First is a freshwater snail, while the second is a freshwater fish.

Habitat: Biliary duct.

Identification: The adult flukes are slender leaf-like and transparent. Generally, the adult flukes are about 7.4 mm in length and 1.5 mm in width, and have two equal suckers, one oral and the other ventral. The digestive system is simple, with a small pharynx and long intestinal ceca. The male testes are two in number, oblique, lobed, and present near the body end. The ovary is slightly lobed, and is located anterior to the testes; the uterus is long and runs anteriorly to open in the genital pore, just above the acetabulum. The vittelline glands present laterally as clusters. The eggs are ovoid shaped and small, about 27-30 µm long and 12-16 µm wide, conatin miracidium when laid, and yellow-brown in color.

Distribution: *O. viverrini* is found mainly in South East Asia, while *O. felineus* is found mainly Europe and in Russia.

Clinical signs are rare but may include symptoms of biliary system dysfunction and affection of the liver.

Control depends on treatment of an infected person with praziquantel, thorough cooking of fish, health education, and good sanitation.

Genus *Clonorichis*
Clonorichis sinensis **(Chinese or Oriental liver flukes).**

Hosts: These are found mainly in humans but other fish eating mammals such as dogs, cats, and rodents are also susceptible. The intermediate hosts are freshwater snails as the first host and freshwater fish as the second host. The life cycle is similar to that of *Opisthorchis* spp. and typically takes about 3 months to be completed.

Habitat: Adult flukes inhabit the biliary ducts, the gall bladder, and occasionally the pancreatic ducts.

Identification: The adult flukes are small (8-25 mm in length by 1.5-5mm in width), and have two suckers, one oral and the other ventral; the latter is smaller than the former. The digestive system is simple, with a muscular pharynx and long, unbranched intestinal ceca. They feature two male testes that are tandem, branched, and present in the posterior one fourth of the body. The seminal vesicle is large. The ovary is located anterior to the testes; the coiled uterus is long and runs anteriorly, opening in the genital pore just above the acetabulum. The vittelline glands present laterally, mainly in the middle third of the worm

Family PARAMPHISTOMATIDAE

Paramphistomes (synonym **amphistomes, paramphistmoids**) is commonly known as "**rumen flukes**" as adult flukes of most species inhabit the fore-stomach (rumen and reticulum) of ruminants. Exceptionally, *Homalogaster paloniae* dwells in the large intestine of bovines. In some species, the adult inhabits the intestinal tract of equines, pigs and humans. One species, ***Explanatum explanatum* (syn. *Gigantocotyle explanatum)***, inhabits the biliary ducts of ruminants in South-East Asia. Their shape is not typical of the trematodes, being conical and fleshy. All are snail-borne trematodes, and require a water snail as an intermediate host.

This family contains several genera, of which *Paramphistomum* is the most common and widespread. The most common species belong to the genus *Paramphistomum*, e.g. *Paramphistomum cervi* and *P. microbothrium*. Other species that may infect ruminants include **Cotylophoron** spp., ***Orthocoelium* (syn. *Ceylonocotyle*) spp., *Calciphoron* spp., *Fischoederius* spp., and *Carmyerius* spp.**

Most species of this family are parasites in ruminants. Species of the genus *Gastrodiscus* infect equids, bovids, elephants and rhinoceros. Other genera such as *Gastrodiscoides* and *Pseudodiscus* infect primates, including human beings, and equids, respectively. Information on the two genera of paramphistomes implicated in human infection is sparse, and concerns mainly species such as **Watsonius watsoni** and *Fischoederius elongatus*, which inhabit the small intestine of humans.

Hosts: Domestic and wild ruminants are hosts for most of these species (see above). Intermediate hosts: Freshwater snails, principally *Planorbis* and *Bulinus*.

Habitat: Adult parasites locate in the rumen and reticulum and immature stages of this parasite locate in the duodenum.

Distribution: The distribution is worldwide. These flukes cause significant economic losses of ruminants, especially in the tropics and subtropics.

Identification of ruminant paramphistomes:
Most species of this family can be readily distinguished from those of other families, because the ventral sucker is at the posterior end of the body, not on its ventral surface. Hence it is called a "posterior sucker". The adults are small, conical, fleshy flukes, about 1-2 cm long. One sucker is visible at the tip of the cone and the other is posterior. The metacercaria, like the adult, has a posterior sucker.

The adult rumen flukes appear as reddish/pink clusters between the papillae of the rumen and reticulum. Adult rumen fluke bodies are thick and fleshy. There are no spines on the cuticular surface. The digestive system begins with an oral opening which leads to a long oesophagus. In most species a pharynx is absent. The intestinal ceca are long and unbranched. There are two testes; the lobated testes are typically in front of the single ovary. The vitellaria are well-developed and usually extend laterally, along the whole length of the body. The uterus is long and coiled, running forwards to the genital pore, in the middle line, in the anterior third of the body. In some species such as *Cotylophoron*, there is an additional sucker, i.e. a "genital sucker", surrounding the genital pore.

The egg resembles that of the *Fasciola* spp., being large, up to 160-180 μm long and 70 μm wide and operculated. The color is clear gray.

Life cycle:
Paramphistomes require an aquatic snail as an intermediate host; the miracidia and larval stages develops in snails of the genera **Bulinus**, **Planorbis** and **Lymnaea**. So the paramphistomes' life cycle is similar to that of *Fasciola*. Under favorable environmental conditions (with temperatures of 26-30°C) the preparasitic developmental stages can be completed within 4-6 weeks.

Eggs pass with the final host feces and hatch in water to produce the miracidium which then penetrates the snail host. There development occurs, yielding sporocysts, redia, and cercariae.

Paramphistomid cercariae are of the leptocercus type (having a simple tail), the body is covered with pigments "***Cercaria pigmentata***" and they have 2 eyespots. Cercariae shed from the snail, encyst on grass and on aquatic plants. After the ruminants ingest the encysted metacercariae on the herbage, the development in the final host occurs in the alimentary tract. Following excystment in the duodenum the young flukes attach and feed there for six weeks before they migrate forward to the fore-stomachs, where they mature into egg-producing adult parasites.

The prepatent period is reported to vary from approximately 56 days in cattle to 70 days in sheep and goats. Adult paramphistomes may survive for many years in the host.

Pathogenesis:
It should be noted that the intestinal immature flukes are more pathogenic than the adults. Further, be it noted that the pathological effects depend mainly on the number of the ingested metacercaria and on the final host species. The pathogenesis of paramphistomiasis can be divided into two phases, the intestinal and the stomach phase.

In the intestinal phase, the size of the immature paramphistomes burden is the most important factor that determines the degree of intestinal damage and the potential clinical effects. Young flukes can cause severe erosions of the deuodenal mucosa. In heavy infections, these cause enteritis, characterized by edema, hemorrhage and ulceration.

Clinically this is characterized by profuse foetid diarrhea (offensive odor) which may be accompanied by anemia, edema and emaciation. Severe cases can lead to death within a few days, especially in young calves and lambs. At necropsy, the young flukes can be seen as clusters of brownish pink parasites attached to the deuodenal mucosa and occasionally to the jejunum and the abomasum.

While in the stomach phase in which the flukes become adult, little if any pathogenic effect is associated with the presence of the flukes in the rumen and/or reticulum, even though large numbers may be present. Localized destruction of rumen papillae may be seen, but this appears to have no significant effect on the host. Adult paramphistomes usually do not cause such severe pathogenic effects except in cases of heavy infection. Then inflammation and erosions of fore-stomach wall can occur.

It should be noted that another species of paramphistomes, i.e. "*Gigantocotyle expalnatum*" develops to maturity in the bile ducts and can cause severe fibrosis and other inflammatory lesions, and clinical signs are similar to that of *Fasciola* spp.

Clinical signs:
The most frequently seen clinical sign of the infection of rumen flukes is diarrhea; usually described as profuse, watery diarrhea with an offensive odor. This diarrhoea may result in anorexia and thirst. In a few cases, hemorrhage can result from long periods of prolonged straining.

Epidemiology:
Paramphistomosis in ruminants results in great economic losses. Endemicity depends on favorable conditions that exist for its snail intermediate host. The infection of cattle, sheep and goats with paramphistomes is very common. These parasites may survive for years, so there is a virtually continual source of reinfection, for successive generations of snails.

The intermediate hosts are extremely adaptable and prolific breeders, which ensure a widespread availability of the snails within the endemic areas. Massive asexual multiplication of the parasites in infected snails and the survival of snails for several months may result in the shedding of large numbers of cercariae.

The disease is more severe in small ruminants at young ages than in large ruminants or in elder animals. Clinical outbreaks of paramphistomiasis are usually confined to the drier months. During this period, the snail population becomes concentrated around natural sources of water. As these areas often provide the only grazing during the dry season, animals may become severely infected. Older animals, especially cattle, seem to acquire immunity to the infection.

Diagnosis:
A diagnosis mainly depends on:
1. Case history (e.g. the snail population in the affected area, the grazing history, etc.)
2. Clinical signs (e.g. profuse, watery diarrhoea with offensive odor)
3. Fecal examination by sedimentation to identify the eggs (but the detection of the eggs occurs mainly in the stomach phase and not in intestinal phase, so such identification may be not significant once the diarrhoea phase has begun).
4. Necropsy procedures.

Paramphistomiasis treatment and control:
Prophylactic therapy can be effective with the use of several drugs, such as "Niclosamide", "Resorantel" and "Oxyclozanide," which are effective against both immature and adult flukes. Methods of controlling parmphistomiasis are similar to control methods for the *Fasciola* species.

Family HETEROPHYIDAE
Genus *Heterophyes*

The family Heterophyidae contains species of both medical and veterinary importance. The most important genus is *Heterophyes*, which contains the most common specie
Heterophyes heterophyes which inhabits the upper intestinal tract of human and fish-eating mammals (canine, feline ..etc). Infection causes severe enteritis, characterized clinically by digestive upset, abdominal pain, and diarrhea.
The life cycle needs three hosts; one definitive vertebrate host and two intermediate hosts. The first intermediate host is a water snail, e.g., ***Pirenella*** spp., while the second intermediate host are fish.

Geographical Distribution: This parasite is found mainly in Egypt, and in the Middle and the Far East.

Identification of *Heterophyes heterophyes*:
The adult flukes are very small and flattened, are about 1-1.7 mm long and 0.3 to 0.7 mm wide, and are of grayish color. The adult flukes have a spiny cuticle, with a characteristic appearance of three suckers (oral, ventral, and genital "gonotyl"). The ventral sucker is larger than the oral one. The digestive system consists of a mouth opening, a long esophagus and unbranched intestinal ceca.
Another morphological mark is the long, coiled uterus that contains the well-developed, small, brown eggs. Two testes are oval, horizontal in position, and present in the posterior one-third of the body. The ovary locates at pre-testicular position. The vitelleria also present laterally in the posterior one-third. Eggs are about 25-30 µm in length, ovoid, with a smooth hard wall, yellow-brown in color, and contain miracidium.

Life cycle of *Heterophyes heterophyes*:
The life cycle comprises three hosts: one definitive vertebrate host and 2 intermediate hosts.
Adults locate between the villi of the upper third of the small intestine. After fertilization, the eggs pass with the feces. They do not hatch until they come in contact with fresh or brackish water. Miracidia swim until they encounter a first intermediate snail host, e.g., ***Pirenella conica***. There it develops into sporocysts and redia, and then into cercariae. The cercariae leave the snail in search of the second intermediate host, which is usually a fish. The cercariae penetrate the fish tissue and develop into the infective stage, the encysted metacercaria. The final host is infected through ingestion of an infected fish. After ingestion, the wall of the cyst is dissolved by the enzymatic action of the hosts' gastric juices in the intestinal tract, and the metacercariae are released and mature.

Pathogenesis of *Heterophyes heterophyes*:
The intestinal flukes are severely pathogenic, due to the spiny cuticle and its minute size. They attach to the intestinal mucosal membrane, especially the upper third of the small intestines (the duodenum) causing severe inflammation i.e., "enteritis". This results in erosion of the intestinal villi. Perforation of the intestine can occur, followed by invasion of the blood and lymph streams, and subsequently other organs can be affected, which may lead to death from heart failure.

Clinical signs of *Heterophyes heterophyes* infection:

The most frequently seen clinical sign is gastric and intestinal upset, abdominal pain, and diarrhea. Fever may also occur, especially if a secondary bacterial infection is part of the clinical picture.

Epidemiology of *Heterophyes heterophyes*:
Heterophyes heterophyes is endemic to certain areas of the world, e.g., Egypt. It is dependent on the availability of hosts (snail, fish, and mammals) and on certain habits of inadequate fish preparation such as poorly salted fish (Fesikh; a traditional home-made salted fish in Egypt).

Diagnosis of *Heterophyes heterophyes* infection:
Diagnosis mainly depends on:

1. Case history (snail population in the area, eating undercooked or poorly salted fish)
2. Clinical signs
3. Fecal examination by sedimentation to identify the eggs.

Treatment and control of *Heterophyes heterophyes* infection:
The best treatment is with the drug praziquantel.
Control depends on:

1. Control of the snail intermediate host.
2. Treatment of infected and carrier humans and animals.
3. Proper preservation, preparation, and cooking of fish
4. Hygienic disposal of human and animal waste.

Genus *Metagonimus*
This parasite infects humans and may infect other fish-eating animals (e.g. dogs, cats, birds). The common species is *M. yokagawai*. It is present mainly in the Far East.

Morphologically, this parasite looks like *H. heterophyes*. The adult flukes are slightly larger than *Heteropheyes* and they typically do not exceed 2.5 mm in length and .75 mm in width. The most prominent feature is the possesion of the acetabulo-gentical apparatus, which looks like a ventral sucker, that is deflected to the right of its midline and that is closely associated with the genital opening. Two testes are large and diagonal to each other, while the smaller ovary is anterior to the testes, and the uterus is filled with eggs. Eggs have a smooth shell, operculated, are yellow-brown in color, ovoid in shape, and small, measuring 28-32 µm in length and 15-17µm in width.

The life cycle, clinical signs, diagnosis, treatment, and control also resemble that of *H. hetrophyes*.

Family ECHINOSTOMATIDAE

Genus *Echinostoma*

These are small, flattened flukes, commonly named "**spiny flukes**", due to the presence of the distinct **spiny head collar** surrounding the oral sucker.

Most members of the genus *Echinsotoma* infect birds, especially aquatic birds, but may also infect rodents, other animals, and humans. Echinostomes inhabit the small intestines.

The geographical distribution of members of the genus *Echinostoma* has a nearly cosmopolitan pattern, but it is more commonly found in Asia, Africa, and southern America.

The most important species are *E. caproni, E. paraensi, E. trivovlus, E. echinatum* and *E. revolutum*.

Identification of *Echinostoma* species:
The adults are small flattened flukes of 5-20 mm long and 2-5 mm wide, elongated, and with a reddish-gray color. Most species have two suckers, a small oral one surrounded by the spiny head collar and a large ventral "acetabulum".

The spines of the collar are usually arranged in one row and 27 or 37 (25-51) in number.

The intestinal ceca are long and straight (i.e. not branched). There are two testes, oval or lobulated in shape and tandem in position. The vitellieria is well developed, lies laterally and extends from anterior to posterior. The single ovary is small, and the uterus is short. It opens into the genital pore, anterior to the acetabulum.

The eggs are small, 90 by 60 μm, straw-yellow in color, and have an operculum.

Life cycle of *Echinostoma* species:
Echinostoma species requires three hosts to complete its life cycle. The adults inhabit the small intestine of aquatic birds, producing eggs which pass with the excreta to the water. The miracidium hatchs from the egg, and searches for the first intermediate host. Snails like ***Physa*** and ***Lymnea*** are a first intermediate host.

After penetration of the molluscan host, the miracidium develops into sporocysts, redia (there are two redial generations, mother and daughter), and then cercariae, which also bear a spiny collar resembling that of the adult. Cercariae shed from the snail search for a second intermediate host, which is usually a tadpole, a fish, or even another snail, where it encysts, forming the infective stage (encysted metacercaria). The infection of the final host occurs through the ingestion of the second intermediate host that contains encysted metacercaria.

Pathogenesis of echinsotomes:
The intestinal flukes are severely pathogenic due to the spiny head collar. They attach to the intestinal mucosa, causing catarrhal enteritis and necrosis of the mucosa.

Clinical signs of echinostomes:
The most prominent clinical sign is diarrhea. Loss of weight and anemia also may be noticed. Deaths may result if a secondary infection occurs.

Epidemiology of echinostomes:
The epidemiology of echinostomes epidemiology is very similar to other snail-borne trematodal infections; it depends mainly on the availability of the hosts and of water. Human infection at present seems to be restricted to Asian countries, depending on food customs, i.e. the opportunity to take undercooked or raw host fish.

Diagnosis of echinostomes:
Diagnosis mainly depends on:
1. Case history.
2. Clinical signs.
3. Fecal examination by sedimentation to demonstrate the eggs.
4. Necropsy to detect and identify the adult flukes.

Treatment and control of echinostomes:
The best treatment is the drug praziquantel.
Control depends on:
1. Control of the snail intermediate host.
2. Treatment of infected and carrier definitive hosts.

Family TROGOLOTREMATIDAE

Genus *Paragonimus*
The most common species is ***P. westermani*** (**human lung flukes**). These flukes infect the lungs of man, cats and many other animals.
The geographical distribution of the *Paragonimus* species is at present confined to the Asia contries.

Identification:
Adult flukes are oval to ovoid in shape. They are small, about 7-12 mm long and 4-6 mm wide, thick, and they are reddish brown in color. They feature two suckers, one oral and one ventral. The intestinal ceca are long and simple. There are two testes, heavily lobulated, horizontal in position, and posterally located. The ovary is also lobulated, much anterior to the testis and on the left side of the median axis of the worm. The vitelline glands are well developed and are located laterally. The eggs are large (about 80-118 μm long and 48-60 μm wide), unsymmetrically ovoid in shape. A marked feature is that the operculum is flattened.

Life cycle:
Adults usually live in a pair, enclosed within a capsule or sacs inside the lungs. After fertizilization, some eggs pass out with sputum or are ingested and pass out with the feces. When eggs reach a water channel, the miracidium develops before being released. The first intermediate host is a snail, while the second is usually a crab. The final host is infected by ingesting the infected crabs containing the encysted metacercaria. After ingestion, the juvenile flukes emerge from the cysts, migrate through the intestinal wall to the peritoneal cavity and then pass through the diaphragm and the pleural spaces to the lungs, where they mature.

Clinical signs of paragonimiasis:
This type of infection may pass unnoticed as the worm burden is typically not high and the worms are encapsulated within the lungs. Clinical signs may include a variety of respiratory manifestations such as a cough and dysponea.

Epidemiology of paragonimiasis:
This parasite is endemic to certain areas of the world, and depends on the availability of hosts (snail, crabs, and mammals) with certain habits of food preparation.

Diagnosis of paragonimiasis:
Diagnosis mainly depends on:
1. Case history such as snail population in the area, whether crabs are available as food.
2. Clinical signs.
3. Sputum and fecal examination to detect and identify the characteristic eggs.
4. Surgical recovery of the worms from the lungs.
5. Radiology diagnosis such as X-ray, CT, MRI etc.

Treatment & control of paragonimiasis:
Although the surgical treatment is of great value, the best treatment is the drug praziquantel.
Control of the parasite depends on:
1. Control of the snail intermediate host.
2. Treatment of the infected carrier, whether human or other animals.
3. Health education
4. Proper preparation and cooking procedure of freshwater crabs.
5. Hygienic disposal of human and animal waste.

Genus *Nanophyetus*
The most common species is *N. slamincola*.
Host: The definitive host is fish eating carnivores, such as dogs and cats. The adult flukes inhabit the small intestines.

Identification:
Adult flukes are small (0.8-2.5 mm long and 0.3- 0.5 mm wide). Tegument is spiny. The oral sucker is slightly larger than the ventral one. The testes are horizontal in position, and located in the posterior third of the body. A small ovary is located just lateral to the ventral sucker and the uterus is short.

Distribution: This species is found in North America.
Like other trematodes, the parasite requires two intermediate hosts; the first is the fresh water snail and the second is fish, particularly salmonids

Pathogenesis and clinical signs:
This worm is thought to be the causative agent of a syndrome called "**Salmon Poisoning**", but it is not. The real causative agent for this syndrome is a rickettsial

pathogen (*Neorickettsia helminthoeca*). However, this flukes transmits the causative agent to dogs and maybe to cats. Salmon poisoning is highly fatal to dogs. Clinical signs of this syndrome include high and persistent fever, diarrhea and vomiting.

Diagnosis of *Nanophyetus* infection:
Diagnosis mainly depends on:
1. Case history.
2. Clinical signs.
3. Examination of the vomit and feces may demonstrate the flukes.
4. Necropsy to detect the flukes that are attached between the intestinal villi.

Treatment and control of *Nanophyetus* infection:
Praziquantel is an effective drug for the parasitic flukes. For the salmon poisoning, condition antimicrobials such as antibiotics and suphonamides are required.

Control depends on:
1. Control of the snail intermediate host.
2. Treatment of the infected carrier hosts.

Family SCHISTOMATIDAE

Members of this family are primarily parasitic in the blood vessels, thus they are called **"blood flukes"**.
The most important genus is ***Schistosoma***, which contains several species of veterinary and medical importance.

Human schistosomiasis (synonym bilhariziasis) is an ancient disease that is very common in some parts of the world (e.g. in Egypt, in the Far East), and is responsible for severe and debilitating conditions.

Hosts:
The final hosts of *Schistosoma* include all domestic mammals. The parasite mainly threatens humans, sheep, and cattle, but can infect other animal species such as pigs, horses, the higher primates, as well as wild ruminants. Water snails are the intermediate host, especially genera ***Bulinus***, ***Biomphilaria***, ***Indopalnorbis***, and ***Oncomelania***. The intermediate snail species differs according to the geographical location.

Habitat:
Schistosoma species infect animals and typically inhabits the mesenteric and intestinal veins; one species "*Schistosoma nasale*" occurs in the nasal veins.

Species:
The major species of this parasite that infect animals include ***S. bovis***, which infects ruminants in Africa, the Middle East, Asia, and southern Europe; ***S. curassoni***, which infects cattle in Africa, ***S. mattheei***, which infects ruminants and occasionally humans in

Africa; and *S. japonicum*, which infects both man and most domestic animals, in the Far East.

Other minor species include *S. leiperi*, which infects cattle in Africa; *S. spindale* and *S. indicum* which infect ruminants, horses, and pigs in Asia; *S. turkestanica* (syn. *Orientobilharzia turkestanica*), which infects ruminants in Asia; and *S. nasale*, which infects ruminants and horses in India and Pakistan.

Human schistomiasis is produced mainly by three species: **S. mansoni, S. haematobium,** and **S. japonicum**.

A form of cutaneous larva migrains called 'swimmer's itch' can occur in man as a result of the cercarial skin penetration (or invasion) of avian (e.g. *Trichobilharzia, Gigantobilharzia*) and animal schitosomes. These migrate in human skin, but do not reach maturity.

Schistosoma identification:
The schistosomes differ from other flukes in that the sexes are separate, the small adult female lying permanently in a groove, **the gynecophoral canal**, inside the body of the male. *Schistosoma* are long, cylindrical (not flattened) flukes, and the tegument bears spines (tubercles).

The sexes are separate in the individual worm; the male, which is shorter and flatter than the female, about 2.0 cm long, and usually carries the thinner female in the gynocophoral canal. These morphological criteria and its habitat site are sufficient for a generic identification. Two suckers are easily seen; a small oral one and a larger, anterior ventral sucker. The digestive system is simple, with no pharynx; the intestinal ceca branch and then they rejoin to form a single canal. In the male, the testes are in the anterior part, and are numerous; they may have as many as nine, in the case of the species cirrus; and its related structures are absent.

In the female, there is a single ovary, the location of which varies according to the species. The egg is large, from 100 - 500 μm long, is spindle-shaped in most species, and it has a lateral or terminal spine. There is no operculum in the egg, and it contains a well-developed miracidium.

The cercaria of schistosomes is called furcocercus cercaria (i.e., a cercaria with a branched tail).

Schistosoma life cycle:
The adults inhabit the blood vessels. After copulation and the formation of the eggs, the female inserts her tail into the smaller blood vessels; there she desposits or pushes in the eggs. Aided by their spines and by the proteolytic enzymes that are secreted by the unhatched miracidia, they then penetrate the endothelium so they can enter the submucosa of the affected tissues.

Then they pass freely through the natural passages (e.g., the intestinal lumen), subsequently they pass of the host with the excreta.

The eggs hatch in minutes in water and their miracidia penetrate the snail, the intermediate host. There the development to the next stage, the cercarial stage, occurs without redial form. There is no metacercarial form. The developmental stages in the snail can be as short as five weeks.

The cercariae actively penetrate the final host via the skin, when the host drinks or otherwise makes contact with contaminated water. After penetration via the skin, the cercariae lose their forked tails, transform to the "schistosomulum stage", as young flukes, and travel via the blood stream through the heart and lungs.
They pass into the systemic circulation and then to the hepatic portal veins. In the liver, these flukes locate in the portal veins and become sexually mature, before they migrate to their final site, the mesenteric veins or pelvis veins.

Schistosoma pathogenesis:

Schistosomiasis or bilhariziasis in humans is both ancient and serious, and threatens human life and welfare. In animals, however, schistosomiasis is considered to be of low veterinary importance.

The major pathogenesis of schistosomes is attributed to their spiny eggs, their habitat as adults, their unusual way of laying eggs, and the toxins that are released as the excretory/secretory products of adult metabolism. These factors independently or together result in an inflammatory and granulomatous response in the affected tissues.

In parts of India to South-East Asia, ***Schistosoma nasale*** infects the nasal mucosal veins of cattle, buffaloes and horses. Severe infections are characterized by mucopurulent discharge, snoring, and dyspnoea (i.e. difficulty in breathing). The main pathogenic effects are associated with the spiny eggs which may cause upper respiratory tract mucosal abscesses. Fibrous granulomatous growths also may occur, which may occlude the nasal passages. Infection is confirmed by the presence of spindle-shaped eggs in the nasal discharge.

Clinical signs and epidemiology of schistosomiasis:

In animals, signs of the disease are rarely seen. In sheep, infection causes anemia and hypoalbuminaemia, with attendant clinical signs that include diarrhea and emaciation. In cattle it can result in low fertility, retarded growth, poor productivity, and death. Outbreaks of bovine schistosomiasis have been recorded in several countries.

There is less data about schistosomiasis in animals than in humans, as researchers have not yet extensively addressed it. Generally speaking, animal schistosomiasis is confined mainly to Africa and Asia. The economic importance of animals schistiomaisis is not yet clear, but is thought to be low. While the prevalence of bovine schistosomiasis seems to be high, the intensity of infection is still low.

Outbreaks of bovine schistoiamsis have been recorded and the occurrence of death in the infected animals. In bovine schistosomiasis, some natural protection, or immunity, against this infection has been observed with aging. The epidemiological factors are similar to that in snail-borne trematodes; in animals the schistosomiasis depends mainly on contact between the susceptible animals and contaminated water with cercariae.

Diagnosis of schistosomiasis:

1. Case history (of low value in animal schistosomiasis).
2. Clinical signs (of low value in animal schistosomiasis).
3. Fecal/urine examination to detect and identify the characteristic spiny eggs. (Note that the tests should be repeated because with advancing age the daily egg output can be low which affects the accuracy of the examination procedure).
4. The serological technique ELISA may be used (which is particularly of good value in human schistosomosis detection, as a way to differentiate between an old and an active infection).
5. Necropsy procedures.

Treatment and control of schistosomiasis:

Praziquantel is the drug of choice in human schistosomiasis; it can also be used in the case of animal schistomiasis. The control is similar to that outlined for other snail-born trematodes, such as **Fasciola** and **Paramphistomum**.

Family DIPLOSTOMIDAE

Genus *Alaria*

The most common species is **A. americana**.

Host: The final host is carnivores (e.g. foxes, wolves, dogs), but this parasite can also affect humans.

Habitat: Adult parasites inhabit the small intestines.

Identification:

Alaria spp. are small flukes with a length of up to 4 mm. A characteristic feature is that *Alaria* body is narrower at the anterior and then widens towards the posterior.

Life cycle:

The life cycle differs from that of other digenetic trematodes, in that it may require at least two intermediate hosts, and as many as four hosts, to complete its life. Adults in the small intestines pass their eggs in the feces, and miracidia are released from the hatched egg and then swim in water until it finds a suitable first intermediate snail host, in which it undergoes development to form a forked tail cercariae. The cercaria leaves the snail and searches for a second intermediate host, which is usually an amphibian, such as a tadpole. In the amphibian host, the parasite develops into the next stage, called the mesocercaria.

The infection of the final host occurs either when it eats the infected amphibian host containing the mesocercariae or when it eats a paratenic host (e.g. snakes) which may harbor the diplostomum as a result of preying on the amphibian host. In the final host, the mesocercaria migrate to the lungs and develop into diplostomum, which then migrate to the intestine and mature.

Pathogenesity:
The adults are quite pathogenic, causing severe enteritis. The infection may be fatal.

4) Class: CESTODA

This class differs from the class Trematoda in that it has a ribbon-like, or tape-like, segmented body so-called "Tape-worms" and no alimentary canal. The body is divided transversely to form separate units, called "segments or proglottids", each mature segment containing one or two sets of genital organs. Cestodes are hermaphrodites. Two orders of veterinary importance are Cyclophyllidea and Pseudophyllidea. Seven important families in Cyclophyllidea are: Taeniidae, Anoplocephalidae, Dilipididae, Davaineidae, Hymenolepididae, Mesocestoididae and Thysanosomidae. One family, Diphylobothridae in the order Pseudophyllidea is of significant veterinary and medical importance

I. Order CYCLOPHYLLIDEA

Structure and function:

The adult cestode consists of a head "also called scolex or holdfast" that bears attachment organs, a short unsegmented neck, and a chain of segments, i.e. "stroblia". The organs of attachment are usually four suckers on the sides of the scolex and these may bear hooks (armed) or not (non-armed). The scolex may have anteriorly a retractable structure called the "rostellum", and in some species this structure may be armed with hooks mentioned above.

The size and the shape of the rostellum is a significant morphological feature for differentiating between genera and species.

The proglottids, also called "segments", bud (i.e., grow) continuously from the neck region and become sexually mature, as they pass down. According to the maturity stage and organs inside, segments can be differentiated into "immature", "mature", and "gravid".

Each mature proglottid is hermaphrotidite, with one or two sets of genital organs. The genital pores typically open on the lateral margin, or margins, of the segment. So the genital openings are either "unilateral" or "bilateral," according to number. Both self-fertilization and cross-fertilization may occur between proglottids. The structure of the genital system is similar to that of the trematodes, i.e., the mature segment contains a male genital system, composed of testes (which vary in number from three up to ten, or even to hundreds, in some species). The testes lead in to a vas deferens, containing the cirrus sac, the seminal vesicle and the cirrus. The female system typically has a single ovary (which may be bi-lobed, tri-lobed or multi-lobed), an oviduct, and the ootype. The vitellierium is present in almost all species, except for a few, e.g., the *Avitellina* spp. As the segment matures and turns to gravid, its internal structure largely disappears and the fully ripe proglottid then contains only a uterus, filled with eggs. The shape of the gravid segment and the uterus within it has a characteristic morphological character to differentiate tapeworm species in some instances. The gravid segments are usually shed intact from the strobila and pass out with the feces.

The eggs are liberated by the breaking down of the segment outside the body.

The egg consists of:

(1) The hexacanth (6-hooked) embryo or onchosphere.

(2) A thick 'shell', called the "embryophore".

(3) A true "egg shell", a delicate membrane which is often lost in excretes.

Cestoda have no alimentary canal. It nourishes by absorption through the tegument. Beyond the tegument, the muscle cells and the parenchyma are found, the latter a syncytium of cells that fill the space between the organs. In the scolex there is a primitive nervous system that consists of ganglia, from which nerves run down to the rest of the body. The excretory system consists of flame cells that lead to efferent canals and these run through the body and discharge at the last segment.

General life cycle of order CYCLOPHYLIDAE:

The typical life cycle of Cyclophylidae is indirect, with one intermediate host, with a few exceptions (e.g. *Rodentolepis nana*). The adult tapeworm is found in the small intestine of the final host, and the gravid segments and the eggs pass in the feces. When the egg is ingested by the intermediate host, the hexacanth embryo is activated. Using its hooks, the embryo migrates through the mucosa to reach the blood or lymph stream or, in the case of an invertebrate intermediate host (e.g. insect), the embryo migrates through the body cavity.

Once in its predilection site, the onchosphere loses its hooks and develops, depending on the species, into one of the larval stages, often known as metacestodes. When the larval stage is ingested by the final host, the scolex attaches to the mucosa, and the remainder of the structure is digested. A chain of proglottids, called as "strobila", begins to grow from the base of the scolex.

Metacestodes of Cyclophylidae:

1. **Cysticercus**. It is best described as a fluid-filled (bladder-like) cyst that contains an attached, single invaginated scolex, sometimes called a "protoscolex" (e.g., *Cysticercus bovis*; the larval stage of *Taenia saginata*).

2. **Coenurus**. It is similar to a cysticercus, but features numerous invaginated scolices (e.g., *Coenurus cerebralis*; the larval stage of *Taenia multiceps*).

3. **Strobilocercus**. It features a scolex that is evaginated and connected to the cyst by a chain of asexual proglottids (e.g., *Strobliocercus fascioliaris*; the larval stage of *Taenia taeniformis*).

4. **Hydatid**. This is a fluid-filled cyst (bladder-like), lined with germinal epithelium, from which invaginated protoscolices are produced in the "brood capsule". The contents of the

cysts (other than the fluid) i.e., the free protoscolices, brood capsules, and their degenerated or necrotic debris can be described as 'hydatid sand'. Occasionally, daughter cysts may be formed "endogenously", completely inside the large cyst, or "exogenously", if the cyst wall ruptures. An example for this metacetsode is, a unicystic hydatid cyst that is the larval stage of *Echinococcus granulosus*.

5. **Cysticercoid**. A single evaginated scolex is embedded in a small solid cyst. It is typically found in an invertebrate, intermediate host such as an arthropod. An example is cysticercoids, those of the family Anoplocephalidae, which form in the body cavity of orbited mites.

6- **Tetrathyridium**. This is a worm-like larva with an invaginated scolex, found only as the larval stage of members of the family Mesocestoididae.

Family TAENIIDAE

This family is of great importance in veterinary science and to public health. The adult tapeworms are found in carnivores and some species may be found in the human small intestine.

Typically, the scolex has an armed rostellum with concentric, double rows of small and large hooks (an exception is Taenia saginata, whose scolex is unarmed). The rostelluar hooks of this family are best described as "dagger or knife-like", with a blade, a guard and a handle. The number and size of the hooks are of significant importance in species identification.

The mature segment is more or less square, with one ovary bilobed. The vitelline glands are present as a compact line mass, just posterior to the ovary. The testes are numerous (from several, to several hundred) and the uterus is simple and sac-like in the mid-line of the segment. The gravid segments are longer than usually their width, and contain the uterus filled with developed eggs.

The eggs, exactly said "embryophore" that contain the hexacanth embryo are small, about 30-40 μm, spherical, and feature double, radially striated walls. The intermediate stage is a cysticercus, strobilocercus, coenurus or a hydatid cyst. These occur only in mammals. In some literatures, the term "bladder worms" is used to describe the metacetodes of the family Taenidae.

Genus *Taenia*

Both the adult and the larval stages of this genus are of importance in human health and in veterinary medicine. The genus contains about 45 species, and these have a worldwide distribution. In the final host, the infection is known as "taeniasis". Infection in the larval stage in the intermediate host can result in "cysticercosis or coenurosis".

The hosts and larval predilection site of the major species of this genus are listed in table 1.

Adult	FH	Larva	IMH	Larval site
T. saginata	Man	Cysticercus bovis	Cattle	Muscles
T. solium	Man	Cysticercus cellulosae	Pig & man	Muscles
T. multiceps	Dog	Coenurus cerebralis	Sheep	CNS
T. hydatigena	Dog	Cysticercus tenuicollis	Sheep	Peritoneum
T. ovis	Dog	Cysticercus ovis	Sheep	Muscles
T. pisiformis	Dog	Cysticercus pisiformis	Rabbit	Peritoneum
T. serialis	Dog	Coenurus serialis	Rabbit	Connective
T. taeniaeformis	Cat	Cysticercus (Strolicercus) fascioliaris	Mouse & Rat	Liver
T. krabbei	Dog	Cysticercus tarandi	Deer	Muscles

Table 1. The final host, larval stage, intermediate host, and the larval predilection site of the Taenia species of major veterinary importance.

Taenia saginata (Beef tapeworm)

The adult tapeworm infects humans where it inhabits the small intestine. The larval stage "Cysticercus bovis" is found in the muscles of cattle, other bovines, though rarely in ovine. This tapeworm is distributed worldwide. Besides its zoonotic importance, it causes considerable economic losses due to infected organ condemnation.

Taenia saginata identification

The length of the adult beef-tapeworm ranges from 5 to 15 or even 20 meters, with an average of 3 to 5. The body consists of several hundreds, up to thousands, of proglottids. The scolex of *T. saginata* has neither rostellum nor hooks (a very characteristic feature). The neck is long and narrow. The mature segment is slightly wider than its length, or is square-like, which is typical for the family. The uterus of gravid segment has approximately 15-20 lateral branches.

The larval stage "Cysticercus bovis" is formed in the striated muscles of the bovine host (e.g. cattle and buffaloes). It is grayish white in color, about 1 cm in diameter, and is filled with fluid, in which the protoscolex is present. It lacks hooks. Cysticercus bovis prefers the heart, the tongue, and the masseter and intercostal muscles.

The life cycle of *T. saginata*

The adult tapeworm inhabits the small intestines of humans. A huge number of eggs (the number may reach in the ten thousands/day) are excreted by the infected person in the feces. These eggs are passed in the feces either individually or within the intact gravid segments. Taenia eggs are resistant to environmental conditions and can survive in feces on pasture for several months.

After the ingestion of *T. saginata* eggs by a susceptible intermediate host, the onchosphere merges and penetrates the intestinal mucosa to reach the blood or lymph stream, where it travels via the blood circulation until it reaches the striated muscle. This stage undergoes development to form the larval stage "Cysticercus bovis", which can be detected in the infected muscles as early as 14 days post infection. It takes about 12 weeks to become fully mature and capable of infecting humans. When C. bovis is fully matured, its diameter is about 1 cm and it is whitish in color, due to the host capsule that surrounds it.

Cysticercus bovis can survive and be infective for several years, but usually old cysts degenerate or become calcified. Man becomes infected by ingesting raw or inadequately cooked meat that contains an infective cyst. It takes two to three months for an infective cysticerus to develop to adulthood.

Taenia saginata pathogenesis, clinical signs

Bovine host does not develop any clinical signs due to cysticercosis. In the human host the adult tapeworm produces a disease condition called "taeniasis" that may not produce symptoms. In some cases, it may produce diarrhea and hunger pains, abdominal pain, nausea, weakness, loss of appetite or increased appetite, headache, constipation, dizziness, anal pruritus, and hyperexcitability.

Taenia saginata epidemiology

A high incidence of *T. saginata* infection has been recorded in many developing countries in Latin America, Africa, and Asia, where there is poor health education, poor sanitation, inadequate food preparation, and where intermediate hosts are plentiful. All these factors enhance the persistence of the *T. saginata* life cycle in humans and in bovine. In developed countries there is a very low incidence of infection from this tapeworm.

Where humans are a final host for *Taenia* species, the infection may be by either *T. saginata* or *T. solium*.

A new species of *Taenia* has been discovered in Southeast Asia, that some literature considers to be a separate species. This is the **Taenia asiatica (the Asian tapeworm)**. Some scholars consider it to be a subspecies of *T. saginata* (i.e., thus ***T. saginata*** *asiatica*). On morphological and genetic grounds, *T. asiatica* resembles *T. saginata* more than *T. solium*. *Taenia asiatica* uses pigs as the intermediate host, and the metacestode localizes in the liver.

Taenia saginata **diagnosis & treatment**

The infection with cysticerci in the bovine host is detected by a routine inspection of carcasses in abattoirs. Inspectors incise and examine various muscles (according to each country's regulations), such as the masseter, and the tongue and heart. The infected part is condemned (a partial condemnation). In the case of numerous numbers of cysticerci in multiple muscles, the whole carcass may be condemned (a total condemnation). There is considerable economic loss to the meat industry.

There are no commercial ante-mortem inspection tests for bovine cysticerciosis nor is there an effective treatment. The drug Praziquantel may be administered twice at a high dose of 50 mg/kg of body weight.

In humans, a diagnosis depends mainly on the detection of taniids eggs or proglottids in feces, as well as on the history and the clinical signs. The drug of choice again is Praziquantel.

Taenia saginata **control**

The control of bovine cysticercosis depends mainly on:

1. Meat Inspection.

2. Health education.

3. Proper disposal of human wastes.

4. Hygienic preparation, preservation, and thorough cooking of meat.

5. Treatment of infected hosts.

Taenia solium

This second species of *Taenia* inhabits the human intestinal tract. The larval stage is called "Cysticercus cellulosae", which develops in the muscles of swine. Interestingly, humans can be the intermediate and the final host for this tapeworm. "Human cysticerciosis" refers to the development of Cysticercus cellulosae within the tissues of an infected person. It is a more serious infection in humans than infection with the adult worm.

Taenia solium identification & life cycle

The morphology of the adult *T. solium* is similar to that of *T. saginata*, with the following exceptions: it is shorter in total length, the scolex is typically of the taeniid type, it is smaller, and has a globular shape. It has a non-retractable rostellum armed with two rows of hooks. The number of hooks ranges from 22-32. The number of testes in the mature segment can reach 200. The uterus in the gravid segment has fewer lateral branches (7-13). The larval stage; Cysticercus cellulosae is about 0.5-1.5 cm in diameter, similar to *C. bovis* but the protoscolex have an armed rostellum.

The life cycle of *T. solium* is similar to that of *T. saginata*, with two exceptions. The intermediate host is primarily the swine, but a human, usually the final host, may also become infected with the intermediate-stage cysticerci; even if this occurs, the life cycle of the parasite is terminated.

Humans may become the intermediate host for *T. solium* either by the accidental ingestion of *T. solium* eggs which may present on foodstuffs contaminated with infected human feces or handled by an infected person, or by autoinfection. Autoinfection can occur by reverse peristalsis, in which the adult tapeworm in the small intestines creates a gastrointestinal disturbance that results in a reverse movement in the gastrointestinal tract. When reverse peristalsis occurs, a gravid segment of the adult *T. solium* may enter the stomach, become ingested by gastric secretion, liberating eggs and oncospheres. The liberated oncospheres then may become activated, migrate through mucosa to the blood stream and so to various organs and tissues, where they develop into C. cellousae.

Taenia solium pathogenesis and clinical signs

As is the case with the *T. saginata* infection, clinical signs in swines are rare to non-existent. In human infection with the adult tapeworm the clinical signs are similar to those of *T. saginata*.

Human cysticercosis manifests various clinical signs, depending on the location of the cysts. Most seriously, cysticerci may develop in the central nervous system and produce clinical signs of nervousness or of mental disturbance. C. cellulosae may also develop in the eye, resulting in ocular cysticercosis, with attendant serious effects on vision. Human cysticercosis is serious zoonoses that affect ten thousands annually, all over the world.

Taenia solium epidemiology & diagnosis

Infection with *T. solium* is not prevalent in the developed countries, and the recorded cases occur when individuals travel to countries where the infection is prevalent. In many developing countries in South America, India, Africa and parts of the Far East this infection is prevalent, although not high. As some religions such as Islam prohibit swine consumption, the disease is very rare among Muslims.

Diagnosis of *T. solium* is similar to that of *T saginata*. In the case of human cysticerciosis, diagnosis depends primarily on serological procedures such as ELISA, that detect the specific antibodies, or by using scanning techniques such as MRI (magnetic resonance imaging) or CT (computerized axial tomography), to locate the cysticerci within the infected organs.

Taenia solium treatment and control

No drug of choice exists now for swine cysticerciosis. In human cysticerciosis, praziquantel and albendazole may be used instead of surgical manipulation. Oxfendazole at a dose 30 mg/kg is shown to be effective.

Control is similar to that given for *T. saginata*.

Taenia hydatigena

A large tapeworm, 120 - 500 cm (average 200) in length, that inhabits the small intestines of the dog and of wild canids. The morphology of this tapeworm is similar to other taenids. The intermediate hosts are mainly sheep and goats; cattle and pigs may be also infected.

The larval stage is "**Cysticercus tenuicollis**" which is a large sac filled with fluid, up to 5-8 cm in diameter, which contains a single invaginated protoscolex. It has a thin wall and is transparent. The predilection sites for C. tenuicollis are the peritoneum and the liver. It may invade other organs. The development from egg to C. tenuicollis takes about four months.

The infection with C. tenuicollis is typically detected at meat inspection. In very rare cases, a condition called "hepatitis cysticercosa" may occur, in which a large number of ingested eggs result in the formation of numerous developed cysticerci that migrate through the liver.

Taenia ovis

This is similar to *T. hydatigena*, with a body length of up to 200 cm. The life cycle is similar to that of *T. saginata*, in that the final hosts are dogs and wild canids. The intermediate stage, **Cysticercus ovis**, is found in the muscles of sheep and goats.

Cysticercus ovis is a small fluid-filled sac, about 1 cm in diameter. The preferred site for C. ovis is the heart, the tongue, and the masseter muscles.

The presence of *T. ovis* cysticerci in the sheep viscera and muscles causes a condition called "sheep measles," which cause considerable economic loss when animals with infected organs are destroyed at meat inspection.

Taenia pisiformis

This tapeworm, up to 200 cm long, inhabits the small intestines of dogs and of other carnivores in its adult form.

The larval stage, **"Cysticercus pisiformis"**, is found on the peritoneum of the rabbit and hare. It is small and pea like, about 1 cm in diameter, and it usually presents in clusters of cysticerci, giving the appearance of a bunch of grapes.

Taenia taeniaeformis

This is a cat tapeworm (i.e., the final host is felines), about 60 cm long. The intermediate stage is **Cysticercus "Stroblicercus" fasciolaris**, which is found in the liver of mice, rats, and other rodents. Each strobilocercus is found within a pea-sized nodule that is partially embedded in the liver parenchyma.

Taenia **(synonym *Multiceps*) *multiceps***

The adult tapeworm is up to 100 cm long and inhabits the small intestines of dogs and of wild canids worldwide. The general morphology is similar to other taenid cestodes. The intermediate hosts include sheep and goats, but the tapeworm rarely infects other ruminants.

The larval stage is **"Coenurus cerebralis"**, which is usually found in the brain of an infected intermediate host.

Coenurus cerebralis is a large, transparent, fluid-filled cyst, up to 5 cm or more in diameter, which breeds clusters of protoscolices on its internal wall.

It takes about eight months for Coenurus cerebralis to develop in the nervous system of the intermediate host. The presence and development of this larval stage results in a syndrome known as "gid or stagger", which is characterized clinically by a circling movement, visual defects, abnormal gait, hyperesthesia (an abnormal increase in sensitivity to stimuli) or paraplegia (an impairment in motor or sensory function of the limbs).

The best treatment is often the surgical removal of the cyst. However for many cases there is no treatment.

Taenia **(syn. *Multiceps*) *serialis***

This is a 70 cm long tapeworm found in dogs. The intermediate stage is "**Coenunrs serialis**", found subcutaneously or in the inter-muscular connective tissue of rabbits. C. seralis is a fluid-filled sac with numerous protoscolices embedded in lines.

Diagnosis, treatment and control of animals with taeniid infection

Diagnosis depends mainly on the demonstration of segments or individual taeniid eggs in the feces. Specific identification of the adult tapeworm is a specialized task of significant research value.

For adult tapeworms, a number of effective drugs are available, including praziquantel, mebendazole, and fenbendazole.

Control depends on breaking the cycle between the intermediate and final hosts through:

1. Treatment of infected dogs/cats.

2. Proper hygienic disposal of dogs/cats feces.

3. Good management practices of the intermediate hosts, to ensure that exposure to the taenid eggs is minimized.

4. The proper hygienic disposal of infected animal meats and offal in abattoirs.

Genus: *Echinococcus*

This is one of the smallest "dwarf" cestodes of domestic animals. This genus includes two main species, *E. granulosus* and *E. multilocularis*. Both are important in veterinary and medical fields. The larval stage, the hydatid, develops in a very wide range of intermediate hosts, including man, and causes a disease called "Hydatid Disease, Hydatidosis or Cystic Echinococcosis".

Echinococcus granulosus sensu lato

E. granulosus is distributed almost worldwide.

Hosts: Mainly dogs and many wild canids, like wolves and coyotes.

Intermediate hosts: Domestic and wild ruminants, humans and swine, as well as horses and donkeys may become infected.

Habitat: The larval stage, "**hydatid cyst**" is found mainly in the liver and the lungs. Adult tapeworms adhere to the mucosa of the small intestine.

Echinococcus granulosus sensu lato identification

The entire cestode is only about 0.5 cm (3-6 mm) long. The tapeworm consists of a scolex and three to five segments. The terminal gravid occupies about half the body length.
Microscopical identification: The scolex is typically taeniid, and bears a taeniid type roestullum, with 28-50 hooks. Each mature segment has a single genital opening with 15-30 testes. The gravid segment contains a branched uterus (with 10-12 branches). The egg is similar to that of *Taenia* spp., and contains a hexacanth embryo in the radially striated embyonophore.

Echinococcus granulosus sensu lato life cycle

The life cycle of *E. garnulosus* is similar to that of other tannids. The adult tapeworm inhabits the small intestines of dogs, and the eggs/gravid segments are passed with the feces. The intermediate hosts ingest the eggs with contaminated food or, frequently in humans, through contamination while playing with infected pet dogs. After ingestion, the onchosphere penetrates the gut wall and travels in the blood to the liver or via the lymphatic system to the lungs.

The liver and lungs are the preferred sites for the unilocular hydatid cyst. Other organs may be infected if onchospheres enter into the systemic circulation and, by this means, breed in other organs and tissues (e.g., the nervous system, spleen, kidney, or bone marrow, etc).

The unilocular hyadtid cyst is a fluid-filled cyst, is opaque and double walled. Its size varies from pea sized to the size of a child's head. Hydatid cysts typically are few, but in some cases, numerous small cysts may develop within the infected organ. The growth of the unilocular hydatid is slow, with maturity in about 6-12 months.

The cyst capsule consists of double layers; an outer thick membrane and an inner germinal epithelium. When cyst growth is almost complete, this epithelium breeds capsules, each containing a number of protoscolices that are budded off. Many of these brood capsules become detached and exist freely in the hydatid fluid. Collectively the contents of broken capsules and the protoscolices are often referred to as 'hydatid sand'. Exogenous or endogenous daughter cysts may be formed from the mother cyst.

Echinococcus granulosus sensu lato pathogenesis and clinical signs

This tapeworm is not pathogenic in dogs and other final hosts. The infection is usually without symptoms. The infection in domestic animals, called "animal hydatidosis", is often detected in abattoirs but not before.

Where onchospheres have been carried in the circulation to other sites, such as the kidney, pancreas, CNS, or marrow cavity of the long bones, pressure from the growing cyst may cause a variety of clinical signs.

However, when humans are an intermediate host, the hydatid in its pulmonary or hepatic site is often of pathogenic significance. One or both lungs may be affected, causing respiratory symptoms, and if several hydatid cysts are present in the liver, there may be gross abdominal distension (i.e., ascites).

Echinococcus granulosus epidemiology

Echinococcus garnulosus is found worldwide; its epidemiological cycle of infection is composed of two cycles, pastoral and sylvatic.

The pastoral cycle always involves the dog, which is infected by feeding on ruminant offal that contains the hydatid cysts. Domestic animals such as sheep and goats typically are the intermediate host, because of their feeding behavior. Other animals that are vulnerable include cattle, buffalo, camels, deer, pigs, and equines. Their vulnerability may be attributed to the close contact between small ruminant herds and the dogs that guard them. This cycle is the main source of cystic echinococcosis infection in humans.

The sylvatic cycle occurs between the wild canids (e.g., wolves and coyotes) and the wild ruminants. This cycle of infection is secondary and of less importance for hydatidosis infection in humans. The pastoral and sylvatic cycles may continue independently or cross each other if domestic dogs become infected through feeding on the viscera of wild ruminants that harbor the hydatid cyst.

Biological and molecular evidence has found many strains of *E. granulosus*, numbered G1 through G10.

The G1 (Sheep strain), G2 (Tasmanian sheep strain) and G3 (Buffalo strain) are called *E. granulosus* sensu stricto. *E. granulosus* sensu stricto strains are the most widespread and the commonest strains involved in cystic echinococcosis infection in animals and humans. The G4 (Equine strain) is *E. equines*. The G5 (cattle strain) is *E. ortleppi*. G6 (camel strain), G7 (Pig strain), G8, and G10 (cervids strain) and of the G9 (uncharacterized host) which may called *E. canadensis*. The other strains such as the lion strain have been found and described. All these strains may be termed *E. granulosus* sensu lato.

Echinococcus granulosus diagnosis

Diagnosis in the final host is very difficult, because of the similarity of *Echinococcus* and *Taenia* eggs. The small size of this tapeworm also makes diagnosis difficult. It can be detected during necropsy procedures.

Other procedures include serological and molecular techniques such as detection of coproantigen and copro-DNA. In the domestic intermediate host, diagnosis of hydatidosis usually occurs during meat inspection at the abattoirs. In humans, diagnosis of cystic echinococcosis depends mainly on serological tests such as ELISA, complement fixation, and immunoelectrophoresis. Scanning techniques (e.g. X-ray, MRI) also are helpful to locate the cyst.

Echinococcus granulosus treatment and control

Praziquantel is effective against adult *E. garnulosus*. Other drugs such as arecoline hydrochloride (purgative anthelmintics) may be used. After administration of the drug it is good to confine the dog to its kennel, to facilitate the collection and disposal of infected feces.

In humans, surgical interference is the primary treatment. Several anthelmintics, such as mebendazole, albendazole, and praziquantel may be used in place of surgery. It should be noted that death from anaphylactic shock may occur during surgical treatment of humans, due to the rupture of the cyst during removal. The formation of daughter cysts is also possible. Surgeons must remove these cysts with great caution.

Control of *E. granulosus* is based on:

1. Maintaining pet dogs on a regular dosage of anthelmintics as a prophylactic treatment and to eliminate any adult tapeworms.

2. Proper disposal of infected animal organs and offal in abattoirs.

3. Control of the stray dog population.

Echinococcus multilocularis

Hosts: Mainly wild canids, but also domestic dogs and cats.

Intermediate hosts: Mainly rodents, such as voles; other animals as well as humans may be infected.

Habitat: The adult parasite occurs in the intestine; the **multilocular hydatid** cyst occurs mainly in the liver.

Distribution: This parasite is found mainly in the Northern hemisphere (e.g., Canada, Alaska, Japan, China, Russia, and some other parts of Europe).

In morphology, it is generally similar to *E. granulosus*, but smaller, with three or four segments. The mature segment can have up to 60 testes. The uterus in the gravid segment is sac-like in appearance.

The life cycle is also similar to that of *E. granulosus*. The larval stage features a "multilocular or alveolar" cyst, which has a diffuse growth, with many compartments that contain a gelatinous matrix into which the scolices are budded off. The alveolar hydatid prefers the liver, where the growth of the intermediate stage is invasive, both extending locally and capable of systemic metastases.

Other species of genus *Echinococcus* include **E. vogeli**, **E. oligoarthus**, and **E. sphiquicus.** These tapeworms are present in the Northern hemisphere and also in Tibet. Wild carnivores and felines are the definitive host in their life cycle. The intermediate host is chiefly rodents. The larval stage of *E. vogeli* and of *E. oligoarthus* is called the **"Polycystic hydatid cyst"**.

Family ANOPLOCEPHALIDAE

Members of this family are the common tapeworms of herbivores.

Genus *Anoplocephala*

The general characteristics of this genus are that they have a scolex with neither a rostellum nor hooks. The mature and gravid segments are wider than they are long. The intermediate stage is a **cysticercoid** that forms in the invertebrate host.

Hosts: Equines e.g., horses and donkeys.

Intermediate hosts: Mites of the family Oribatidae.

Habitat: The adult tapeworm is found in the small and large intestine, and the cysticercoids are found in forage mites.

Species: *Anoplocephala perfoliata* and *A. magna*.

Distribution: Worldwide, *A. perfoliata* is more common.

Anoplocephala **identification**: *A. magna*, *A. perfoliata*, and *Paranoplocephala mamillana* are the only adult cestodes commonly found in equines. A rare cestode infection of the genus *Moniezia*, *M. palida*, has been recorded in equines in South Africa and India.

Anoplocephala perfoliata is a large white fluke, up to 20 cm in length, with a rounded scolex with a lappet behind each of the four suckers. It features a very short neck and the strobila widens rapidly. The individual proglottids are much wider than they are long.

Anoplocephala magna is similar morphologically but is much longer, up to 80 cm in length. There are no lappets on the scolex. The eggs are irregular, spherical, or triangular and vary from 50 to 80µm in diameter. The onchosphere is supported by a pair of projections called the pyriform apparatus.

Anoplocephala life cycle

The mature segments are passed in the feces and then disintegrated, releasing the eggs. The eggs are ingested by the intermediate host mites, in which in 2-4 months they develop to the cysticercoid stage. One or two months after the ingestion of the infected mites within the herbage, the adult tapeworm is found in the intestine of the final host.

Anoplocephala pathogenesis

Anoplocephala species is usually non-pathogenic but in the case of heavy infection it may cause severe clinical signs and even prove fatal. *Anoplocephala perfoliata* is usually found around the ileo-cecal junction and causes ulceration of the mucosa. These lesions are a cause of intussusception, which is usually fatal in horses. *A. magna* is more commonly found in the jejunum and when present in large numbers may result in catarrhal or haemorrhagic enteritis. Cases of intestinal obstruction and perforation of the intestinal wall have been recorded and usually results in death.

Anoplocephala clinical signs and epidemiology

Infection with *Anaplocephala* is usually symptomless. But loss good body condition, a rough coat, enteritis, and colitis may be observed.

Anoplocephala diagnosis, treatment and control

Diagnosis and treatment depends mainly on the demonstration of eggs (contain the characteristic pyriform apparatus) on fecal examination.

Pyrantel is the drug of choice in the treatment of *Anoplocephala* infection in equines. Control depends mainly on prophylactic anthelmintics treatment.

Genus *Paranoplocephala*

The most commom species is ***Paranoplocephala mamilliana***.

Paranoplocephala mamilliana is the third species of adult tapeworm that can infect equines. It is usually non-pathogenic. It is a small tapeworm, up to 5cm long and 0.5cm wide.
It inhabits the duodenum and sometimes the stomach of horses in most parts of the world.
There are no lappets on the scolex and the suckers are slit-like. The life cycle is similar to that of *Anoplocephala* spp.

Genus *Beritella*

Members of genus *Beritella* are parasites of the small intestines of primates and rodents, marsupials, and may also infect humans. Mites are thought to be the intermediate host for these cestodes.

Genus *Moniezia*

This genus of cestodes is common in ruminants.

Hosts: Ruminants.

Intermediate hosts: Mites, mainly of the family Oribatidae.

Habitat: Adults locate in the small intestine; cysticercoids locate in mites.

Species:
Moniezia expansa infects mainly sheep, goats, and occasionally cattle,

M. benedeni infects mainly cattle, sheep, and goats.

M. alba infects mainly sheep and other ruminants

M. trigonophora infects mainly camels and other ruminants

M. palida infects mainly equines

Distribution: Worldwide.

***Moniezia* identification**

These are long tapeworms, up to 2 meters or more in length.

The scolex is small, globular, and without hooks. It possesses four cup-shaped suckers. Mature segments are broader than they are long and contain two sets of genital organs grossly visible along the lateral margin of each segment. The tapeworm can have 140 to 160 testes. The two ovaries are lateral with each followed by vitelline glands. There are two large genital pores.

There is a row of interproglottidal glands at the posterior border of each segment which may be used in species differentiation.

In *M. expansa* these extend along the full breadth of the segment. In *M. benedeni* they are confined to a short, continuous row, close to the middle of the segment. In *M. alba* the interproglottidal glands are absent. In *M. trigonophora* the testes are arranged in a pyramidal shape around the ovaries. In the gravid segment of *Moniezia* spp., the internal structure disappears with the exception of the uterus which forms a large sac that occupies most of the segment and is filled with eggs.

The eggs can be triangular or quadrate or irregular in shape. They have a well-defined pyriform apparatus and vary in size from 55 to 75µm in diameter.

Moniezia life cycle

This is similar to *Anoplocephola*. The mature proglottids or eggs are passed in the feces and the onchospheres are ingested on pasture by forage mites. The embryos migrate into the body cavity of the mite, where they develop to cysticercoids in 1-4 months. Infection of the final host occurs by ingestion of the infected mites during grazing.

The prepatent period is about 6 weeks.

Moniezia pathogenesis

Usually the infection is symptomless, but in severe infection it can cause poor condition, diarrhea, and even intestinal obstruction.

Moniezia clinical signs and epidemiology

Infection usually occurs with no clinical signs. Infection is more common in young animals than in older animals.

Moniezia diagnosis, treatment and control

Diagnosis is based largely on the presence of mature segments and of characteristic eggs in the feces, or detection of adult worms at necropsy or at the abattoir. The drugs niclosamide and praziquantel can be used for treatment. Control seems difficult, but routine treatment of the animals and rotation of the pasture may help.

Family THYSANOSOMIDEA

Genus *Stilesia*

The most common species is *Stilesia hepatica*. Infection with this tapeworm is common in sheep and other ruminants in Africa and Asia.

Adults inhabit the bile ducts.

The length of the adult tapeworm varies from 20-50 cm. The scolex has no rostellum and the suckers are unarmed. The proglottids are narrow and wider than they are long. A mature segment contains a single set of genital organs and a uterus bilobed. The two lobes of the uterus are connected with a transverse bar. The mature eggs pass into a paruterine organ. Each gravid segment contains two such paruterine organs. The paruterine organ is a thick shell sac-like structure formed as a result of evagination of the uterine wall. When fully mature, the structure detaches from the uterus and forms a thick walled capsule around the eggs.

Clinical signs of this infection are rare.

The eggs possess a pyriform apparatus and the intermediate host is probably an orbited mite.

Stilesia globipunctata, another species, occurs in the small intestine of ruminants in southern Europe, Africa, and Asia.

Treatment is rarely required, but praziquantel is effective.

Genus *Thysanosoma*

The most common species is *Thysanosoma actinioides* which known as "**fringed tapeworm**" since each segment has a row of large, grossly visible papillae along the posterior border of each segment.

Like *S. hepatica*, it is found in the bile ducts of sheep and other ruminants. The economic impact is largely condemnation of the liver at meat inspection. Its geographical distribution is confined to North and South America.

The adult cestode measures up to 30cm in length. The mature segment contains a double set of genital organs. The gravid segment has a well-developed paruterine organ. The intermediate host is thought to be the orbited mite or bark lice.

Niclosamide has shown to be an effective drug.

Genus *Avitellina*

Avitellina centripuctata is the common species that found in the small intestines of sheep, cattle, camels, and other ruminants in southern Europe, Africa, and Asia. This tapeworm resembles *Moniezia* species except that it is narrower and the segmentation is poorly marked so that it appears somewhat ribbon-like.

It may reach up to 3 meters in length. The scolex has no rostellum or hooks. The mature and gravid segments are narrow and broader than they are long. The mature segment contains a single set of genital organs, with a centrally located uterus.

When the eggs form, they pass to a thick shell, paruterine organ.

This tapeworm has little pathogenic effect.

The intermediate hosts are thought to be oribitid mites or bark lice.

Treatment is the same as that for *Thysanosoma*.

Family DILEPIDIDAE

Genus *Dipylidium*

Species: ***Dipylidium caninum*** **(Cucumber tapeworm, Double-pore tapeworm)**

Hosts: Dogs and cats. Rarely found in humans.

Intermediate hosts: Fleas (mainly *Ctenocephalides canis* and *C. felis*) and lice (*Trichodectes canis* and *Heterodoxus spiniger*).

Habitat: Adult found in the small intestine; cysticercoids are found in fleas and lice.

Distribution: Worldwide

Dipylidium caninum **Identification**

An adult *D. caninum* is about 30-50 cm in length; the scolex has four suckers and a contractible rostellum, which is armed with four or five rows of small hooks. The mature and gravid segments are shaped like a cucumber seed, are elongated, and have two sets of genital organs, with two genital pores opening on each lateral margin. The gravid segments are active, and can crawl about on the tail region of an animal. The onchospheres are contained in egg packets or capsules, each containing approximately 20 eggs.

Dipylidium caninum **life cycle**

Cysticercoids develop in the body cavity of the intermediate host (i.e., fleas, lice), which takes the eggs. Note that all stages of the dog louse can ingest onchospheres. But the adult flea, with its mouthparts adapted for piercing, cannot. In fleas the infection is acquired during the larval stage, which has mouthparts adapted for chewing. The development from onchosphere to cysticercoid in the dog louse occurs more quickly than in fleas.

The final host is infected by ingestion of the flea or louse that contains the cysticercoids. The prepatent period is about 3 weeks.

Dipylidium caninum pathogenesis, clinical signs and epidemiology

The adult tapeworm is usually non-pathogenic to the infected animals, with no clinical signs. But some cases may exhibit abdominal discomfort and diarrhea. In humans, the infection may pass without clear symptoms. Children are more susceptible than adults particularly if they play with pet animals.

Dipylidium caninum is a very common infection in dogs and cats all over the world. Stray dogs and cats play an important role in maintaining the cycle, as domestic pets usually have routine anthelmintics and insecticide treatment.

Dipylidium caninum diagnosis

Diagnosis depends mainly on the detection of the characteristic gravid segment in the feces or around the anal opening. Diagnosis also depends on the demonstration of the egg packets in a fecal examination.

Dipylidium caninum treatment and control

In a *Dipylidium*-infection the infected animal should be treated with both anthelmintics and insecticide; the dog house should be thoroughly cleaned and sanitized. The administration of anthelmintics such as praziquantel should be accompanied by the use of insecticides like malathion or diazinon.

The animal's bedding and rest areas should be treated with insecticides to eliminate the immature stages of the flea.

Genus *Amoebotaenia*

The most common species are *A. cuneata* (syn. *A. sphenoides)*

This is a dwarf tapeworm that occurs in domestic chickens and that may infect other birds.

It inhabits the small intestines.

This tapeworm is up to 4 mm long, but consists of several proglottids, as many as 30. It is more or less triangular in shape.

The scolex bears armed rostellum with 12-14 hooks and unarmed suckers. The mature segment contains a single set of genital organs. The intermediate stage, a cysticercoid, is usually found in earthworms. It is not normally pathogenic unless present in very large numbers.

Genus *Choanotaenia*

Choanotaenia infindibulum

This is a large tapeworm found in chickens. The worm is about 20 cm in length, and is white in color.

The scolex has an armed rostellum with 16-22 large hooks and four unarmed suckers. A mature segment contains a single set of genital organs, the ovary is central, and there may be as many as 60 testes. These are concentrated in the posterior portion of the segment. Each segment widens towards the posterior, giving the margin of the tapeworm a 'saw-edge' appearance. The eggs are filamentous.

The life cycle is indirect. The cysticercoid may be found in the house fly, *Musca domestica*, and in beetles.

Information about its pathogenicity is scanty.

Family DAVAINEIDAE

Genus *Davainea*

Davainea proglottina is the most common species. It is a very pathogenic cestode found in poultry.

Distribution: It is distributed worldwide.

Hosts: Domestic fowl and pigeons.

Intermediate hosts: Slugs and land snails.

Habitat: The adults are found in the small intestine; the cysticercoids are found in slugs and snails.

Davainea proglottina identification, pathogenesis and control

This is a small cestode (dwarf) up to 4 mm long; its body consists of 6-9 segments. Both the rostellum and the suckers bear hooks. Severe infections may cause hemorrhagic enteritis, due to the hooks in the rostellum and suckers. A light infection may cause retarded growth and weakness. Both infection and signs of infection are more prominent in young birds. Control depends on treatment of the infected birds with anthelmintics such as niclosamide and the destruction of intermediate slugs and snails wherever possible.

Genus *Raillietina*

This genus includes numerous species that are mainly parasitic in birds.

The most important species **is *Raillietina echinobothrida***. These are up to 25cm long and feature a rostellum with numerous hammer-shaped hooks and four armed suckers. The mature segment has a single set of genital organs and a central ovary. The testes are numerous and are scattered around the ovary. The gravid segments have eggs packed in egg capsules.

In severe infections, the embedded scolices of this parasite in the mucosa produce large caseous nodules in the wall of the small intestine. Signs include diarrhea, weakness, and emaciation.

The life cycle is indirect. Ants and beetles serve as the intermediate hosts.

Other common species include **R. *tetragona*** and **R. *cesticillus*.**

Control depends on anthelmintics to treat the *Davainea* and insecticides to destroy the intermediate hosts.

Family HYMENOLEPIDIDAE

Genus *Rodentolepis*

Members of this family, which has a characteristically slender strobila, infect birds, rodents and humans. The intermediate form is a cysticercoid.

Rodentolepis (= Hymenolepis) nana is the common tapeworm in humans and also in rodents.

It is of interest in that the life cycle can be direct as well as indirect.

The cysticercoids develop in the villi of the small intestine of the final host and then emerge to develop into the adult tapeworm. This is about 30 mm long and is found in the intestinal lumen. Flour beetles or fleas may serve as an intermediate host in the indirect transmission.

Rodentolepis nana **identification**

The adult *R. nana* scolex bears s retractable rostellum armed with 20-30 hooks and four suckers. The scolex is followed by a long, narrow neck. The mature and gravid segments are wider than they are long, the genital pores are unilateral, and each mature segment contains three testes and one central ovary. The gravid segment is also broader than it is long and it contains a sac-like uterus filled with eggs. The eggs are small 30-46μm in diameter and have filaments on both poles of the embryonophore.

Rodentolepis nana life cycle

The life cycle of *R. nana* is exceptional in that it can be direct (with no need for an intermediate host) or indirect (utilizing a flea or a beetle as an intermediate host).

In the direct life cycle, infection occurs through ingestion of eggs, which are transferred in contaminated food. The eggs hatch in the duodenum, releasing oncospheres, which penetrate the mucosa and come to lie in the lymph channels of the intestine.

The oncospheres develop into a cysticercoid; after 5-6 days the cysticercoids emerge into the lumen of the small intestine, where they attach and mature into adults. In the indirect life cycle, the cysticercoid is formed in the flea or beetle, and the infection occurs through consumption of foodstuffs contaminated with infected fleas or beetles.

The cysticercoids then emerge in the intestinal lumen and attach to form an adult. The infection is more common in children than in adults. The symptoms include weakness, change in appetite, and occasionally toxemia.

A diagnosis depends mainly on demonstration of the characteristic eggs in the feces. The drugs praziquantel or niclosamide are the treatment of choice. Control depends on health education, improvement of personnel hygiene, and early treatment of infected individuals.

Hymenolepis diminuta or "**rat tapeworm**" is the common tapeworm found in rats worldwide but these rarely infect other animal hosts or humans. This tapeworm is much similar to *R. nana*, but differs in its morphology, being larger, up to 20-60 cm in length. The scolex has no rostellum and the eggs lack a filament.

The life cycle is indirect. It uses only beetles as its intermediate host.

Other species of *Hymenolepis* are recorded in domestic poultry (e.g., ***Hymenolepis carioca, H. lanceolata,* and *H. anatina***). These are of no public health importance and of low veterinary importance.

Genus *Fimbriaria*

The most common species is **Fimbriaria fasciolaris**, which is an unusual tapeworm found in ducks, geeses, and chickens and may also affect other birds. In ducks it is large (up to 43 cm long). It also occurs in chickens. The most characteristic morphological feature is the flaring anterior neck region, which is known as the pseudoscolex. The scolex has smooth suckers and a retractible arm. The intermediate host is a crustacean such as *Cyclops*.

Family MESOCESTODIDAE

These cestodes infect carnivorous animals and birds. There is little information about the members of this family.

It is generally thought to have two metacestode stages. The first stage is a cysticercoid, found in an insect or mite; the second is a solid larval form, a **tetrathyridium**, found in a vertebrate.

Habitat and distribution:

The adult cestodes are found in the small intestine of dogs, cats, and wild carnivores in parts of Europe, Asia, Africa, and North America. They are up to 40 cm in length, each segment having a central genital pore. The unarmed scolex has four suckers.

The life cycle of the parasite apparently requires two intermediate stages in two hosts. The first intermediate stage is a cysticercoid in a host mite and the second is a tetrathyridium in the peritoneal or pleural cavity of a wide variety of vertebrates. They are of veterinary interest because a dog or cat may be the definitive host and these animals may also host tetrathyridia in their peritoneal cavity. These tetrathyridia, each 1.0 cm or longer, have the capacity to multiply asexually and the resulting massive infections may produce severe ascites in an infection with *M. vogeli*.

Order PSEUDOPHYLLIDEA

The morphology of Psudophyllidea is different than that of the Cyclophyllidea, as the scolex has no suckers but two longitudinal grooves or bothria.

The egg shell is thick, light brown, and operculate. The egg emerges from genital pore in the mature/gravid segment. They hatch in water.

The larval stages are the "**coracidium**", a motile ciliated onchosphere with an embryophore. This coracidium develops into a "**procercoid**" in the first intermediate host, which is usually a crustacean organism such as "*Cyclops*". The last larval stage is the "**plerocercoid**" stage which develops in the muscles and the viscera of the second intermediate host, a water organism such as fish and amphibian. The plerocercoid is the infective stage for the final host; it is a solid structure, about 5 mm in length and has a characteristic scolex.

Family DIPHYLOBOTHRIDAE

Genus *Diphylobothrium*

Diphylobothium latum **"broad fish tapeworm"** is the longest tapeworm that can infect humans.

Distribution

This species is distributed worldwide, particularly in Europe, the Scandinavian countries, Russia and North America. In Asia, ***D. nihonkaiense*** is involved in human infection.

Hosts: Man and fish-eating mammals such as the dog, cat, wild carnivores, and bears. Intermediate hosts: Crustacean organisms such as Cyclops are the first intermediate host; the second is the freshwater fish.

Identification: The adult is very long, up to 10 meters in length, and may contains 3000 segments. The scolex is unarmed, with two muscular longitudinal grooves "bothria" as organs of attachment, instead of suckers (i.e. no suckers, no hooks).

The mature and gravid segments are wider than they are long, with a central genital pore. The mature segment contains a rosette-shaped uterus filled with eggs when gravid. The eggs are yellow in color. The ovary is bilobed. The vitteliera and the testes are distributed in most parts of segments, in close conjunction. The eggs are continuously discharged from the genital pores of the attached gravid segments of the strobila and pass to the exterior with the feces.

The eggs resemble that of the *F. hepatica* eggs and are yellow in color and operculate, but are approximately half the size (about 70 μm in length).

Diphylobothrium latum life cycle

The eggs hatch in water within a few weeks to liberate a motile ciliated coracidium. The procercoid is developed within the *Cyclops* that feeds on the coracidium. The plercoercoid develops in the muscles and viscera of fish that have fed on the infected *Cyclops*. The final host becomes infected from ingesting a raw or undercooked fish containing the plercoercoid.

The prepatent period is about four weeks.

Diphylobothrium latum pathogenesis, clinical signs, control and treatment

In humans, *D. latum* may cause intestinal symptoms, but the main sign is a macrocytic anemia, resembling pernicious anemia, due to its uptake of vitamin B_{12} from the intestine. In some regions of the world, the dried adult *D. latum* was once used as a treatment of anemia, due to its richness in vitamin B_{12}.

Humans are the main host for *D. latum*. Its epidemiology depends mainly on the access of human sewage to freshwater channels and the ingestion of uncooked fish. Other animals can play a role in maintaining the cycle as a final host.

Diagnosis depends mainly on the detection of the characteristic eggs in the feces by sedimentation (care must be taken to not confuse the eggs with those of *Fasciola* spp.).

Praziquantel and niclosamide are effective treatment drugs.

Control depends mainly on hygienic disposal of human sewage and good preservation and cooking of fish.

Genus *Spirometra*

Adult *Spirometa* are found in the intestinal tract of dogs, cats, and wild carnivores.

The morphology and life cycle of these tapeworms is similar to that of *D. latum*. The first intermediate host is a crustacean and the second is an amphibium, a bird or a mammal. Humans can be infected either by consumption of drinking water containing procercoid-infected crustacea or from eating a plerocercoid-infected host.

This tapeworm is responsible for a disease in humans, known as sparganosis, derived from the name Sparganum for the plerocercoid. Sparagnosis has been found in Southeast Asia, where the muscles of snakes and frogs have been used as traditional medicine for wounds, and in the human diet.

Clinically the disease is characterized by the presence of the plerocercoid in the muscles and subcutaneous tissues, particularly the periorbital area, causing edema and inflammation.

REFERENCES AND SUGGESTED READINGS

Ballweber L R (2001). The practical veterinarian. Veterinary Parasitology. Butterworth–Heinemann publications. Library of Congress Cataloging-in-Publication Data.

Cui J, Lin X-M, Zhang H-W, Xu B-L, and Wang Z-Q (2011). Sparganosis, Henan Province, Central China. Emerging Infectious Diseases 17(1): 146-147.

De Bont J and Vercruysse J (1997). The Epidemology and control of cattle schistomiasis. Parasitology Today, 13 (7): 255-262.

Denegri G, Bernadina W, Serrano J P and Rodriguez-Caaberio F (1988). Anaplocephalid cestodes of veterinary and medical significance: a review. Folia Parasitologica, 45:1-8.

Dewey, S. 2001. "*Hymenolepis diminuta*" (On-line), Animal Diversity Web. Accessed March 24, 2014 at http://animaldiversity.ummz.umich.edu/accounts/Hymenolepis_diminuta

Eckert J, Gemmell M A, Meslin F-X and Pawłowski Z S (2001). WHO/OIE Mannual on Echinococcosis in Humans and Animals: a public health problem of global concern. World Organisation for Animal Health (Office International des Epizooties) and World Health Organization, 2001 Reprinted: January 2002, World Organisation for Animal Health, Paris, France. ISBN 92-9044-522-X.

Eduardo S L (1982). The toxonomy of family Paramphistomatidae Fischoeder, 1901 with special reference to the morphology of species occuring in ruimnants. I. General Consideration. Systematic Parasitology, 4:7-57.

Grove D I (1990). A history of human helminthology. CAB International, Wallingford. UK: 848 pp. OIE Terrestrial Manual (2008). CYSTICERCOSIS: 1216-1226.

Hodgson, E. and E. Knapp 2003. "*Dipylidium caninum*" (On-line), Animal Diversity Web. Accessed March 24, 2014 at http://animaldiversity.ummz.umich.edu/accounts/Dipylidium_caninum.

Jang D H (1969). Study on *Eurytrema pancreaticum* II. Life Cycle. The Korean Journal of Parasitology, 7 (3): 178-200 (In Korean language with English summary).

Kasny M, Beran L, Siegelova V, Siegel T, Leontovyc R, Berankova K, Pankrac J, Kostakova M and Horak P (2012). Geographical distribution of the giant liver flluke (*Fascioloides magna*) in Czech Republic and its potential risk of its further spread. Veterinarni Medicinia, 57 (2): 101-109.

Kaupp, B.F. (1918). Animal parasites and parasitic diseases. Third Edition. Alexander Eger. Available at http://www.archive.org/details/cu31924056979226.

Khalil LF, Jones A and Bray R A (1994). Keys to cestode parasites of vertebrates. First Edition, CAB International.

Le T H, Nguyen V D, Phan B U, Blair D and McMannus D P (2004). Case report: Inusual presntation of *Fasciolopsis buski* in a Vite Namese child. Transactions of the Royal Society of Tropical Medicine and Hygiene, 98: 193-194.

Lloyd J, Boray J and Love S (2007). Primefact 452, Stomach Fluke (*Paramphistomes*) In Ruminants. First Edition, Department of Primary Industries, New South Wales Government, Australia, available at http://www.dpi.nsw.gov.au/agriculture/livestock/health/specific/cattle/stomach-fluke-ruminants

Lotfy W M and Hillyer G V (2003). *Fasciola* species in Egypt. Experimental Pathology and Parasitology; 6: 9-22.

Macpherson C N L, Gottstein B and Geerts S (2000). Parasitic food-borne and water-borne zoonoses. Rev. sci. tech. Off. int. Epiz.,19 (1), 240-258.

Mas-Coma S and Bargues M D (1997). Human live flukes: A review. Reserach and Reviews in Parasitology, 57 (3-4): 145-218.

Manga-Gonzalez M Y, Gonzalez-Lanza C, Cabanas E and Campo R. (2001). Contributions to and review of dicrocoeliosis, with special reference to the intermediate hosts of Dicrocoelium dendriticum. Parasitology, 123: S91-S114.

Marinculiæ A, Džakula N, Janicki Z, Hardy Z, Luèinger S and Živiènjak T (2002). Apperance of American liver fluke (*Fascioloides magna*, Bassi, 1875) in Croatia- a case report. Vetreinarski Archiv 72 (6): 319-325.

McDougald L R (2011). "Cestodes and trematodes". In Saif Y M, Fadly A M, Glisson J R, McDougald L R, Nolan L K, Swayne D E. Diseases of Poultry (12 Edition). Iowa (US): Blackwell Publishing Company. pp. 1057–1066.

McManus D P, Zhang W, Li J and Bartely P B (2003). Echinococcosis. Lancet, 362:1295-1304.

Murell K D (2013). Zoonotic foodborne parasites and their surveillance. Rev. sci. tech. Off. int. Epiz., 2013, 32 (2), 559-569.

Nakao M, Lavikainen A., Iwaki T, Haukisalmi V, Konyaev S, Oku Y, Okamoto M and Ito A (2013). Molecular phylogeny of the genus *Taenia* (Cestoda: Taeniidae): Proposals for the resurrection of *Hydatigera* Lamarck, 1816 and the creation of a new genus *Versteria*. International Journal of Parasitology, 43: 427-437.

OIE Terrestrial Manual (2008). Chapter 2.1.4- Echinococcosis/Hydatidosis. Pp 175-189.

Olson P D, Criba T H, Tkach V V, Bray R A and Littlewood D T J (2003). Phylogeny and classification of the Digenea (Platyhelminthes: Trematoda). International Journal for Parasitology, 33:733–755.

Otranto D. and Traversa D. (2002) A review of dicrocoeliosis of ruminants including recent advances in the diagnosis and treatment. Veterinary Parasitology 107: 317–335.

Otranto D and Traversa D. (2003). Dicrocoeliosis of ruminants: a little known fluke disease. Trenes in Parasitology, 19 (1): 12-15.

Otranto D and Traversa D. (2002). A review of Dicrocoeliosis of ruminants including recent advances in the diagnosis and treatment. Veterinary Parasitology, 107: 317-325.

Roberts L S and Janovey J (2009). Gerald D. Schmidt & Larry S. Roberts—Foundations of Parasitology. Eight Edition, McGraw-Hill Comp., NY. USA. Chapters 13- 21; pp: 201-367.

Romig T, Dinkel A and Mackenstedt U (2006). The present situation of echinococcosis in Europe. Parasitology International, 55:S187-S191.

Sanabria R E F and Romero J R (2008). Review and update of Paramphistomosis. Helminthologia, 45 (2): 64-68.

Solusby, E.J.L. (1982): Helminths, Arthropdes, and Protozoa of Domesticated Animals. 7th Ed. Baillier, Tindal and Cassel, London.

The center of food and security and public health, Iowa state University (2011). Echinococcosis. Available at www.cfsph.iastate.edu/Factsheets/.../echinococcosis.pdf

Thompson R C A (2008). The taxonomy, phylogeny and transmission of Echinococcus. Experimental Parasitology, 119:439-446.

Urquhart G M, Armour J, Duncan J L, Dunn A M and Jennings F W (1996). Veterinary Parasitology. Second Edition, Blackwell Science Ltd.

Vitta A, Srisawangwong T, Sithithaworn P, Laha T and Tesana S (2004). Laboratory production and maintenance of *Spirometra erinacei* spargana. Southeast Asian Journal of Tropical Medicine and Public Health, 35, Sup.1: 280-283.

Yamaguti, S. (1958). Systema Helminthum. Volume I. The digenetic trematodes of vertebrates. Part I and II. Interscience Publisher, INC., New York.

Yamaguti, S. (1959). Systema Helminthum. Volume II. The Cestodes of Vertebrates. Interscience Publisher, INC., New York.

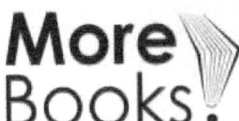
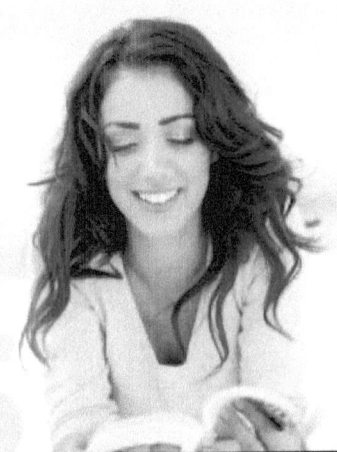

I want morebooks!

Buy your books fast and straightforward online - at one of world's fastest growing online book stores! Environmentally sound due to Print-on-Demand technologies.

Buy your books online at
www.morebooks.shop

Kaufen Sie Ihre Bücher schnell und unkompliziert online – auf einer der am schnellsten wachsenden Buchhandelsplattformen weltweit! Dank Print-On-Demand umwelt- und ressourcenschonend produziert.

Bücher schneller online kaufen
www.morebooks.shop

KS OmniScriptum Publishing
Brivibas gatve 197
LV-1039 Riga, Latvia
Telefax +371 686 204 55

info@omniscriptum.com
www.omniscriptum.com

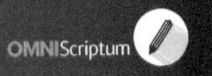

www.ingramcontent.com/pod-product-compliance
Lightning Source LLC
Chambersburg PA
CBHW031545210526
45464CB00003B/1155